Bendix

English for Qualified Medical Employees

Englisch für Medizinische Fachangestellte

2. Auflage

VERLAG EUROPA-LEHRMITTEL · Nourney, Vollmer GmbH & Co. KG
Düsselberger Straße 23 · 42781 Haan-Gruiten
Europa-Nr.: 79558

Autor: Heinz Bendix, 91629 Weihenzell

2. Auflage 2015, korrigierter Nachdruck 2021

Druck 5 4 3 2

Alle Drucke derselben Auflage sind parallel einsetzbar, da sie bis auf die Behebung von Druckfehlern unverändert sind.

ISBN 978-3-8085-7998-5

www.europa-lehrmittel.de
Umschlaggestaltung: Tiff.any GmbH, 10999 Berlin
Satz: Punkt für Punkt GmbH · Mediendesign, 40549 Düsseldorf
Druck: RCOM Print GmbH, 97222 Würzburg-Rimpar

VORWORT

Dieses Buch ist für Medizinische Fachangestellte im Berufsschulunterricht konzipiert.

Es setzt die durch einen qualifizierenden Hauptschulabschluss bzw. durch die Mittlere Reife erworbenen Englischkenntnisse voraus. Eine Wiederholung der englischen Grammatik ist daher nicht vorgesehen.

Schwer zu merkende, sprachlich und grammatikalisch komplizierte Ausdrucksweisen werden vermieden.

Die Satzkonstruktionen sind so einfach wie möglich, aber dennoch korrekt.

Da die Lernenden bereits im Beruf stehen, sollte die vom Rahmenlehrplan geforderte kommunikative Kompetenz im Umgang mit Englisch sprechenden Patienten in möglichst kurzer Zeit erreicht werden.

Aufgrund der bei allen Auszubildenden bereits vorhandenen Kenntnisse der englischen Sprache und deren Grammatik kann auf allzu kleinschrittiges Vorgehen weitgehend verzichtet werden. Die Auszubildenden sollten von Anfang an grundsätzlich an das Sprechen in **vollständigen** Sätzen gewöhnt werden.

Dieses Buch dient als intensiver Aufbaukurs in fremdsprachlicher Kommunikation, wobei auf Übungen verzichtet wird, die wertvolle Unterrichtszeit beanspruchen und doch die geforderte kommunikative Kompetenz nur wenig fördern.

Sprechkompetenz erwirbt man nur durch ständiges Sprechen. Da dies im Unterricht aus Zeitgründen leider nicht allen Lernenden gleichzeitig möglich ist, sollten **sämtliche** Dialoge, Fragen und Antworten grundsätzlich **von allen** Auszubildenden einer Klasse **schriftlich** formuliert werden. Dieses Vorgehen ist zwar mit erheblichem Aufwand verbunden, verbessert die Sprechkompetenz und die Nachhaltigkeit des Erlernten jedoch ganz entscheidend.

Das Buch ist kompakt und beschränkt sich auf wichtige Grundübungen. Den Lehrpersonen steht es frei, ihren Unterricht auf der Grundlage dieses Buches durch eigene kreative Ideen zu bereichern, falls sie dies für notwendig halten.

Hinweis: Im britischen Englisch ist ein Punkt hinter Abkürzungen wie z. B. Ms (Miss), Mrs (Mistress) oder Mr (Mister) nicht mehr üblich. Im amerikanischen Englisch wird er jedoch weiterhin verwendet.

Die **2. Auflage** entspricht der vorherigen und wurde lediglich an einigen Stellen korrigiert.

Verlag und Autor wünschen Ihnen viel Erfolg bei der Arbeit mit *English for Qualified Medical Employees.*

Autor und Verlag im Frühjahr 2015

INHALTSVERZEICHNIS

1 AT THE SURGERY OF A GENERAL PRACTITIONER

Michael and Karen Brady, an American couple, moved to Germany some time ago. Back home in the States, Mrs. Brady worked as a medical assistant at a medical center for about five years. Kathrina is a qualified medical employee. She works at the surgery of the general practitioner Dr. Astrid Kessler and takes every opportunity to speak English. Kathrina already knows the Bradys. It is Friday, 6 o'clock in the afternoon. She is meeting Mrs. Brady on her way home from work ...

Mrs. Brady Hi, Kathrina. Nice to see you! How are you doing?

Kathrina Hello, Mrs. Brady. I'm fine, thanks. But I'm so glad it's Friday!

Mrs. Brady Oh, how come?

Kathrina It has been such a stressful week ...

Mrs. Brady Really? Well, I know what you are talking about. Did I tell you that I worked as a medical assistant at a medical center back home in the States? I did that job for more than five years. I worked as a receptionist. What do you have to do at your doctor's office?

Kathrina Well, I mainly sit at reception. As I'm in direct contact with the patients I have to do a lot of talking all day long. Welcoming the patients, giving them advice, sending them to the different rooms in our surgery, taking care of patient files, answering phone calls, making appointments, writing prescriptions, sick certificates, doctor's letters and lots more is my job. My colleague Eva calls me the "computer expert" because I know our surgery administration program inside out. As the German health system keeps changing frequently, our software provider sends us software updates whenever there are any changes. And the changes are very frequent, you know! That's why my colleague Eva is much better off.

Mrs. Brady Better off? Why?

Kathrina She doesn't have to do so much talking and has to do less administrational work. My colleague Eva is our "lab expert". She takes blood specimen, makes electrocardiograms, does pulmonary function tests and Dr. Kessler even allows her to put up intravenous drip infusions, to give injections or to vaccinate. Before she vaccinates, she usually checks the patient's certificates of vaccination. She is very experienced as she has been doing her job for more than twenty years now.

Mrs. Brady Do you also have to assist Dr. Kessler?

Kathrina Sometimes. But it is mainly Eva who assists Dr. Kessler when she is with a patient in the treatment room. She helps her when Dr. Kessler has to stitch a cut, has to dress a wound or needs any other medical assistance.

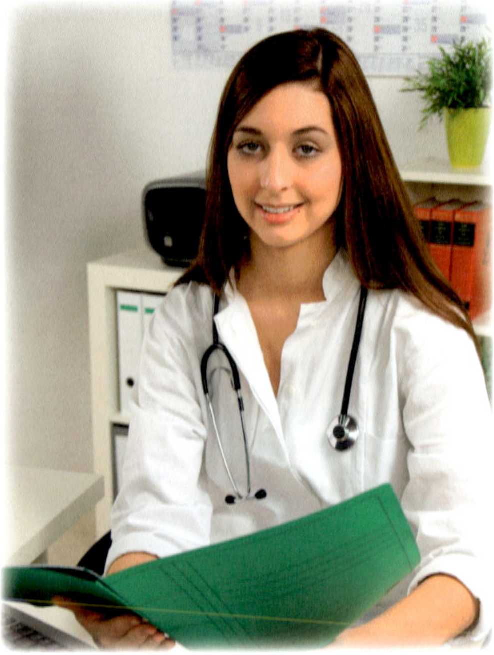

Mrs. Brady Do you make X-rays in your office?

Kathrina We make ultrasound scans but we don't make X-rays. For X-rays we send our patients to a radiologist ...

ACTIVITY 1

Please note ...

It is advisable to make your own list of unknown words and expressions. You should know every word and every expression before doing the other exercises in this book. Vocabulary work never is a waste of time and should be done as an essential part of every lesson! Do the vocabulary work in pairs or in groups. Now, find the following words and expressions in the text and make your own, personal vocabulary list! (Work from left to right.)

Words in the texts, which you do not find here, you will find in the vocabulary list at the end of each unit.

Arztpraxis (UK)	Facharzt/-ärztin für Allgemeinmedizin	umziehen, ziehen
vor einiger Zeit	daheim in den Staaten (USA)	Medizinische Assistentin
Ärztehaus, MVZ	Medizinische Fachangestellte	jede Gelegenheit ergreifen
auf dem Nachhauseweg	Wie geht es Ihnen?	Danke, gut.
Ich bin froh ...	Wieso?, Warum? (Slang)	stressig
hier: MFA, welche an der Anmeldung arbeitet	Arztpraxis (UK)	an der Anmeldung, am Empfang, Rezeption
jemanden begrüßen	Rat geben	sich kümmern um
Patientenakten	Anrufe entgegennehmen	Termine ausmachen
Rezepte schreiben o. drucken	AU-Bescheinigung	Kollege, Kollegin
Praxisverwaltungsprogramm	in- und auswendig	jedoch
Software Anbieter	häufige Aktualisierungen	Gesundheitssystem
es ändert sich ständig	deshalb	sie ist „besser dran“
Laborexpertin	Blut abnehmen	Lungenfunktionsprüfung
hier: legen	intravenös	Tropfinfusion
impfen	Impfbücher überprüfen	sehr erfahren sein
assistieren, helfen	Klar! Sicher!	hauptsächlich
Behandlungsraum	nähen	Schnittwunde, schneiden
verbinden	Wunde	Röntgen
röntgen (Verb!)	Ultraschalluntersuchung	Radiologe

DAS SOLLTEN SIE WISSEN ...:

Surgery heißt eigentlich „Chirurgie“. Das Wort ***surgery*** wird im britischen Sprachraum jedoch nicht nur für die Chirurgie, sondern auch für die Arztpraxis als Ganzes wie auch für die Räume innerhalb einer Arztpraxis (Sprechzimmer, Behandlungsraum usw.) verwendet. Im amerikanischen Sprachraum spricht man dagegen nicht von doctor's ***surgery***, sondern von doctor's ***office*** (Arztpraxis), bzw. dentist's or dental ***office*** (Zahnarztpraxis). Die in Deutschland verwendete Bezeichnung „Facharzt für Allgemeinmedizin“, entspricht im britischen wie auch im amerikanischen Sprachraum der eines ***general practitioner***. Er wird im Allgemeinen kurz als ***GP*** bezeichnet, lässt sich aber eher mit den bei uns noch tätigen „Praktischen“ Ärzten vergleichen. Die Praxis eines GP nennt man ***general practice***, manchmal auch ***general surgery***, obwohl dieser Begriff auch für „Allgemeinchirurgie“ steht. Ein „Arzt“ ist in englischsprachigen Ländern ein ***physician***. Jedoch werden Ärzte dort, wie auch in Deutschland, gewöhnlich als „doctor“ bezeichnet, auch wenn sie keinen Doktortitel besitzen. „Doctor“ ist ein von einer Hochschule verliehener akademischer Titel und keine Berufsbezeichnung. Ein ***physician*** bzw. ein Arzt muss, wie Sie sicher wissen, nicht notwendigerweise einen Doktortitel führen um eine Zulassung als Arzt (Approbation) zu erhalten. Ein „Hausarzt“ wird übrigens ***family doctor*** or ***family physician*** genannt.

UNIT 1

ACTIVITY 2

Please, answer the following questions in English!

1. When did Mrs. Brady move to Germany?
2. How long did she work at a medical center in the States?
3. What job did she have back home in the States?
4. What is Kathrina's job?
5. Kathrina says: "I'm so glad it's Friday". Why does she say that?
6. Where does Kathrina mainly sit when she is at work?
7. Kathrina thinks that her job is very stressful. Why does she think that?
8. Which are the different things Kathrina has to do when she is at work?
9. Everybody calls her the "computer expert". Why?
10. Kathrina is convinced that her colleague Eva is much better off. What makes her think so?

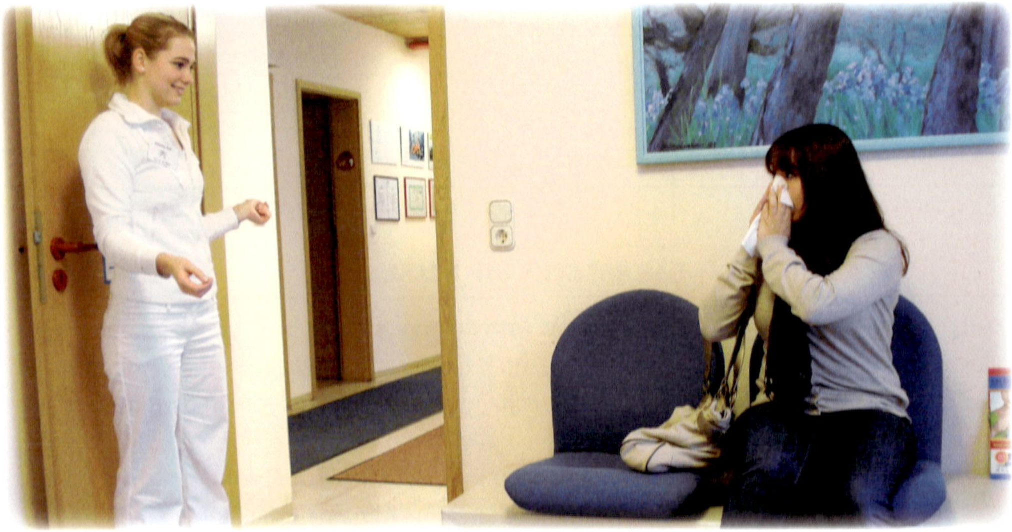

ACTIVITY 3

All these statements are false. Please correct them!

1. Mrs. Brady worked at the surgery/at the office of a neurologist.
2. Dr. Astrid Kessler is a dentist.
3. Back home in the States Mrs. Brady worked as a medical assistant for about fifteen years.
4. Kathrina mainly works in the laboratory.
5. Dr. Kessler has not got a laboratory.
6. Dr. Kessler does all injections, infusions and vaccinations herself.
7. For ultrasound scans patients are sent to a radiologist.

ACTIVITY 4

Can you say it in English!

1. Ich zog von Köln nach Berlin um.
2. Ich arbeitete 15 Jahre lang als MFA in Köln.
3. Ich arbeitete in der Praxis einer Allgemeinärztin.
4. Bist du auch eine MFA?
5. Frau Dr. Kessler ist Fachärztin für Allgemeinmedizin.
6. Wir sollten jede Gelegenheit nutzen, um Englisch zu sprechen.
7. Es war eine stressige Woche.
8. Hallo, wie geht's?
9. Oh, mir geht es gut.
10. Ich weiß, wovon Sie sprechen.
11. Daheim in Alabama arbeitete ich in einem Medizinischen Versorgungszentrum.
12. Sitzt du auch an der Anmeldung?
13. Ich mag es, in direktem Kontakt mit den Patienten zu sein.
14. Ich muss den Patienten oft Rat geben/erteilen.
15. Ich kümmere mich um die Patientenakten.
16. Ich nehme Anrufe entgegen.
17. Ich mache Termine aus.
18. Kann ich bitte ein Rezept haben?
19. Ich habe zwei Kolleginnen.
20. Das Praxisverwaltungsprogramm ändert sich ständig.
21. Mit dem deutschen Gesundheitssystem ist es genauso.
22. Eva, die oft im Labor ist, ist viel besser dran.
23. Sie hat nicht so viele Verwaltungsarbeiten zu erledigen.
24. Ich darf auch intravenöse Infusionen legen.

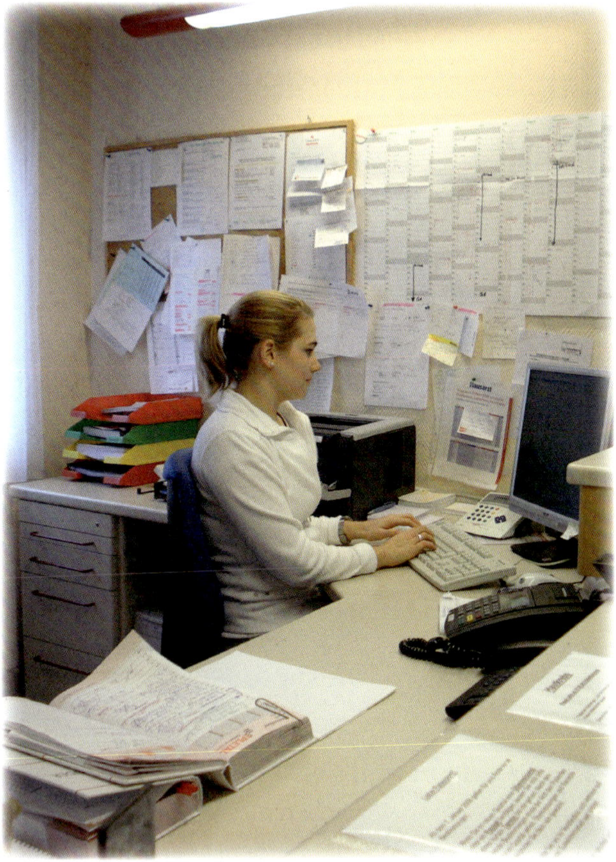

25. Sie nimmt Blut ab, verabreicht Spritzen, impft und führt Lungenfunktionsprüfungen durch.
26. Wir sind sehr erfahren.
27. Wir machen auch EKGs.
28. Manchmal muss ich Frau Dr. Kessler assistieren.
29. Ich bin oft im Behandlungsraum.
30. Frau Doktor Kessler wird Ihre Schnittwunde nähen.
31. Danach werde ich Ihre Wunde verbinden.
32. Wir machen Ultraschalluntersuchungen, aber kein Röntgen.
33. Zum Röntgen schicken wir unsere Patienten zu einem Radiologen.
34. Ich benötige eine Arbeitsunfähigkeitsbescheinigung für meinen Arbeitgeber (employer).
35. Haben Sie Ihr Impfbuch dabei (with you)?

ACTIVITY 5

Have this conversation in English with one of your colleagues in class!

Colleague	Was für eine Ärztin ist Frau Dr. Kessler?
You	Sie ist Ärztin für Allgemeinmedizin.
Colleague	Röntgt ihr auch?
You	Nein, aber wir machen EKGs, Ultraschalluntersuchungen und Lungenfunktionsprüfungen.
Colleague	Was machst du häufig?
You	Ich bin oft im Labor und nehme Blut ab. Ich verabreiche Spritzen, darf impfen, lege intravenöse Infusionen und assistiere, wenn ein Patient im Behandlungsraum ist. Und du?
Colleague	Ich sitze häufig an der Anmeldung, nehme Anrufe entgegen, mache Termine aus, schreibe Rezepte, AU-Bescheinigungen, Arztbriefe und vieles mehr. Ich kümmere mich auch um die Patientenakten.
You	Verwendet ihr auch schon das neue Praxisverwaltungsprogramm?
Colleague	Ja, seit zwei Monaten. Ich kenne das neue Programm schon in- und auswendig.
You	Habt ihr auch Patienten, die nur Englisch sprechen?
Colleague	Manchmal, aber nicht sehr oft. Und ihr?
You	Wir haben einige Englisch sprechende Patienten. Die meisten von ihnen sind Amerikaner die in der US-Armee dienen (serve).

ACTIVITY 6

Now, ask your neighbour questions in English. Take turns!

Ask her/him ...

1. ... if she/he often works at reception.
2. ... how long she/he has been working as a medical assistant.
3. ... if she/he has to work in the lab.
4. ... what she/he usually does there.
5. ... if she/he already knows the surgery administration program very well.
6. ... if she/he has direct contact with the patients.
7. ... if she/he sometimes has to assist the doctor.

Doctor: **What seems to be the trouble?**

Patient: **After I get up in the morning, I always feel sick for half an hour.**

Doctor: **Then why don't you get up half an hour later?**

(seem = scheinen; trouble = Beschwerden, „Welche Beschwerden haben Sie denn?"; get up = aufstehen; feel sick = sich krank/übel fühlen)

ACTIVITY 7

Have a conversation with a partner!

You	Partner
1. Begrüßen Sie Ihren Partner/Ihre Partnerin.	
	2. Erwidern Sie etwas.
3. Sie fragen, wie es ihm/ihr geht.	
	4. Sie antworten, dass Sie froh sind, dass es Freitag ist, weil die Woche sehr stressig war.
5. Sie möchten wissen, warum die Woche so stressig war.	
	6. Sie erklären warum und sagen ihr, dass es Ihre Arbeitskollegin viel besser hat.
7. Sie möchten wissen, inwiefern sich Ihre Arbeit von jener Ihrer Arbeitskollegin unterscheidet.	
	8. Sie schildern die unterschiedliche Aufgabenverteilung in Ihrer Praxis

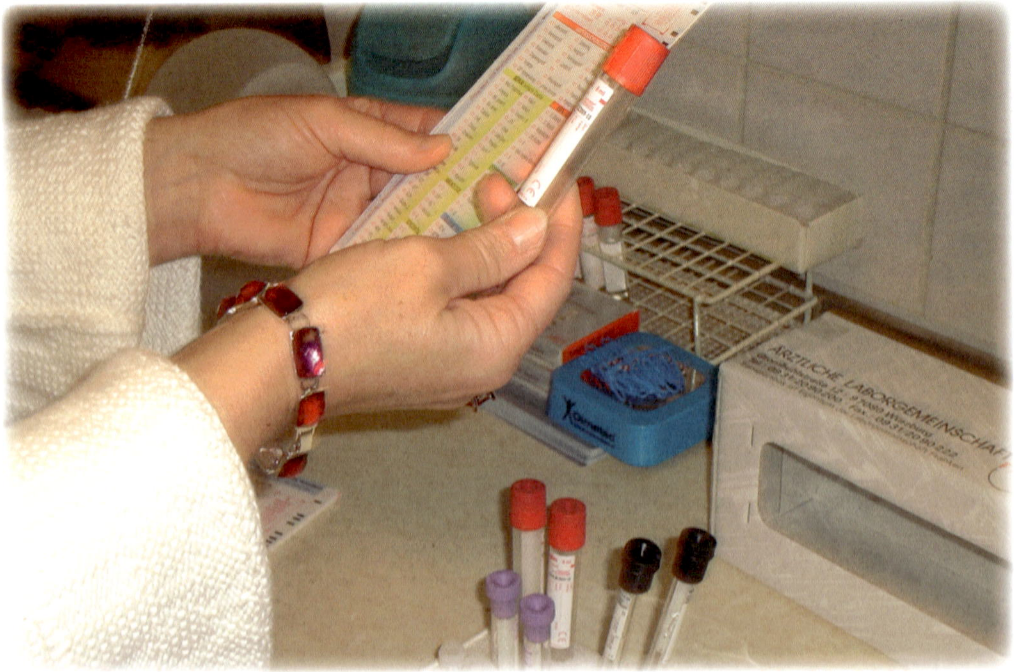

EXTENDED VOCABULARY LIST	
administration	Verwaltung
advice	der Rat
advisable	empfehlenswert, ratsam
advise	raten, Rat geben
along with	zusammen mit
assist	helfen, assistieren
busy	voll, beschäftigt
certificate **sick certificate** **certificate of vaccinations („shot record“)**	Bescheinigung AU-Bescheinigung Impfbuch; (Hinweis: jede Art von Injektion oder Impfung, wird gewöhnlich als „shot“ bezeichnet).
colleague	Kollege, Kollegin
convinced	überzeugt
doctor's letter	Arztbrief
enter	eintreten, betreten

essential	wesentlich, lebensnotwendig
experienced	erfahren, sachkundig, versiert
expression	Ausdruck, Redewendung
extended	erweitert
false	falsch, unwahr
few	wenige, einige
file	Akte, Datei
frequent	häufig
general	allgemein
glad	froh
How come?	Wieso? (Umgangssprache)
mainly	hauptsächlich
neurologist	Neurologe
opportunity	Gelegenheit
part	Teil
prescription	Rezept, Verschreibung
provider	Anbieter
qualified employee	Fachangestellte/r
reception (desk)	Anmeldung, Reception, Anmeldetheke
record card	Karteikarte
specimen/sample	Probe, Muster
scan	abtasten, überfliegen; hier: Ultraschalluntersuchung
sick certificate/sick note	AU-Bescheinigung
stitch	Stich, Seitenstich, nähen
surgery	die Praxis, die Chirurgie
take care (of)	kümmern (um)
take turns	sich abwechseln
treatment	Behandlung
to vaccinate	impfen
waste **surgery waste** **waste of time**	Abfall, Müll Praxisabfall Zeitverschwendung
wound	Wunde

2 MEDICAL SPECIALISTS IN GERMANY

Kathrina's English teacher at school asked her to give a short lecture in English to the class. The topic of her lecture is: "Survey of the Different Medical Specialists in Germany". This is what she wrote ...

"Physicians who are not specialized are called ***general practitioners*** or, as the people also call them, ***GPs***. Doctors who treat the ear, the nose and the throat are so called ***ENT specialists***. ENT stands for: **E**ar, **N**ose and **T**hroat. ***Gynaecologists*** treat diseases of women or women expecting a baby. If someone has got a problem with his or her kidneys, sexual organs or his or her urinary bladder, then the person needs to see a specialist, who is called a ***consultant urologist***. In Germany, you would call such a specialist "Facharzt für Urologie". People also call those doctors ***urologists***. Heart specialists are called ***cardiologists***. If a doctor needs further information on what is happening inside the body, the doctor may refer the patient to a ***radiologist***. For the diagnosis of diseases the radiologists use very expensive equipment. They do computer tomography (CT), magnetic resonance imaging (MRI) or X-ray. If a patient has got a skin problem or suffers from an allergy, he or she has to see a ***consultant dermatologist***. An ***internist*** specializes in internal diseases. The internist will examine the lungs if a patient has a breathing problem or problems with the stomach, gastro-intestinal system, liver, gallbladder or other organs. It may happen that a person has broken bones, has a walking problem, has a damaged or slipped disc or a meniscus problem, then the patient should see (also: consult) an ***orthopaedist***. Doctors who are specialized in children's diseases are called ***paediatricians***. If patients have got problems with their eyes, need contact lenses or glasses, the patients will have to see an ***oculist*** that is an eye specialist. Doctors, who treat diseases of the nervous system, are called ***neurologists***. Doctors, who mainly work at hospitals and do operations, are called ***surgeons***. There are medical consultants who specialize in the medical field of *oncology*. That is the diagnosis and treatment of malignant tumours. Those specialists are called ***oncologists*** or ***cancer specialists***".

ACTIVITY 1

Find these words and expressions in the text and add them to your personal vocabulary list!

einen Vortrag halten	Thema	Überblick, Übersicht
Allgemeinarzt	behandeln	Hals, Rachen, Kehle
HNO-Arzt	Frauenarzt	Krankheit
Frauenleiden, Frauenkrankheiten	erwarten	Harnblase
Nieren	Geschlechtsorgane	aufsuchen, sehen
Facharzt für Urologie	Urologe	Kardiologe
weitergehende Informationen	innerhalb	überweisen, weiterleiten
Radiologe	Diagnose	teuer
Ausrüstung, Ausstattung	Computertomografie	Kernspintomografie, MRT
Röntgen	leiden an	Allergie
Hautarzt	Internist	Krankheiten der inneren Organe
untersuchen	Lunge	Atembeschwerden
Magen	Darm	Leber
Gallenblase	Es könnte passieren	Knochen
Knochenbruch	Gangbeschwerden	verletzte Bandscheibe
Bandscheibenvorfall	Meniskus	Orthopäde
Facharzt für Orthopädie	Kinderkrankheiten	Kinderarzt
Kontaktlinsen	Brille(n)	Augenarzt
Nervenkrankheiten	Neurologe	Facharzt für Neurologie
hauptsächlich	Operationen	Chirurg
medizinisches (Fach-) Gebiet	Onkologie	bösartig
Geschwulst	Onkologe	Krebsspezialist

Surgeon to patient: I'm afraid we have to operate you again because I forgot my rubber gloves inside you.

Patient: I'd rather pay for them if you just leave me alone.

(rubber gloves = Gummihandschuhe; I'd rather = Ich würde lieber; to pay for them = sie zahlen; to just leave someone alone = jemanden einfach in Ruhe lassen)

UNIT 2

UNIT 2

ACTIVITY 2

Give an answer in English!

Ask her/him ...

1. What was the topic of Kathrina's lecture?
2. Who asked her to give the lecture?
3. What kind of doctor is a GP?
4. What does "ENT" stand for?
5. What diseases does a consultant gynaecologist treat?
6. In which cases would you visit a consultant urologist?
7. What kind of specialists are cardiologists?
8. In which case would a GP refer a patient to a radiologist?
9. What do radiologists do to diagnose diseases?
10. Which doctor would you consult if you suffer from a skin problem?
11. Which diseases does an internist specialize in?
12. Give a few examples of organs which internists usually examine!
13. In which cases do patients consult an orthopaedist? Give examples!
14. Which doctors are specialists for the treatment of children's diseases?
15. In which cases would a patient visit an oculist?
16. Which diseases do neurologists specialize in?
17. Which doctors would you often find at hospitals?

ACTIVITY 3

Can you say it in English!

1. Dr. Meyer ist Chirurg und arbeitet auch im Krankenhaus.
2. Er operiert dort.
3. Ich arbeite in einer kardiologischen Praxis.
4. Er ist leidet an einer schlimmen Krankheit.
5. Morgen gehe ich zur Frauenärztin.
6. Viele Menschen haben Probleme mit ihrer Niere oder der Harnblase.
7. Es ist am besten, wenn Sie einen Urologen aufsuchen.
8. Sie erwartet ein Kind.
9. Wir überweisen Sie zu einem Onkologen.
10. Wir denken, es ist eine Erkrankung Ihres Nervensystems.
11. Wenn Sie Kontaktlinsen oder eine neue Brille brauchen, müssen Sie einen Augenarzt aufsuchen/konsultieren.
12. Meine Tochter hat Masern. Morgen suche ich einen Kinderarzt auf.

13. Ich habe seit zwei Wochen Atembeschwerden.
14. Gehen Sie zu einem Internisten, der auf Lungenerkrankungen spezialisiert ist!
15. Ich bin zu einem Orthopäden gegangen.
16. Ich dachte, ich hätte mir mein Bein gebrochen.
17. Man hat mein Bein geröntgt.
18. Es sind keine Knochen gebrochen.
19. Ich habe immer noch Beschwerden beim Gehen.
20. Der Arzt meint, es sei der Meniskus.
21. Ich habe seit Sonntag Rückenbeschwerden.
22. Kann es ein Bandscheibenvorfall sein?
23. Gestern war ich beim HNO-Arzt.
24. Wenn Sie allergisch sind, sollten Sie zum Hautarzt gehen.
25. Radiologen sind wichtig, um Krankheiten zu diagnostizieren.
26. Wegen meiner Hautprobleme hat man mich zu einem Facharzt überwiesen.
27. Haben sie Probleme mit Ihrem Hals, Ihrer Nase oder Ihren Ohren? Dann sollten Sie einen Hals-, Nasen-, Ohrenarzt aufsuchen.

Frank L. Morrisson MD
Consultant Paediatrist

Consulting hours:	Mon – Wed	8 am to 4 pm
	Thu	8 am to 12 am
		3 pm to 6 pm
	Fri	8 am to 11 am

Phone 01706 377 599

Patient: Doctor, you've got to help me. I just can't stop my hands from shaking!

Doctor: Do you drink a lot?

Patient: Not really – because of my shaky hands I spill most of it!

(to stop = aufhören; shake = schütteln; shaky = zittrig; spill = verschütten)

ACTIVITY 4

Have a conversation with a partner in your class!

You	Partner
1. Wie nennt man in Englisch sprechenden Ländern einen Arzt, der nicht spezialisiert ist?	
	2. Ärzte, die nicht spezialisiert sind, nennt man dort Allgemeinärzte.
3. Ein Internist ist ein Facharzt für welche Erkrankungen?	
	4. Er ist Facharzt für innere Krankheiten und ist spezialisiert auf Erkrankungen der inneren Organe wie Lunge, Magen-Darm-Trakt, Gallenblase, Leber und Bauchspeicheldrüse.
5. Kümmert er sich auch um Nieren, Harnblase oder Geschlechtsorgane?	
	6. Nein, bei Erkrankungen dieser Organe sucht man einen Urologen auf.
7. In welchen Fällen sucht man einen Augenarzt auf?	
	8. Wenn man an einer Augenkrankheit leidet, Kontaktlinsen oder eine Brille benötigt.
9. Dein Allgemeinarzt ordnet eine CT oder MRT bei dir an. Zu welchem Arzt wird er dich überweisen?	
	10. Zu einem Radiologen.
11. Welchen Facharzt suchst du auf, wenn du Probleme mit deinen Bandscheiben, deinen Menisken oder deinen Knochen hast?	
	12. Ich suche einen Orthopäden auf.
13. Was ist ein „Neurologe“?	
	14. Ein Facharzt/Spezialist für Erkrankungen des Nervensystems.
15. Eine Frau erwartet ein Kind. Welchen Facharzt sollte sie aufsuchen?	
	16. Einen Frauenarzt.
17. Was ist (eigentlich) ein „Onkologe“?	
	18. Ein Onkologe diagnostiziert und behandelt Tumore.

EXTENDED VOCABULARY LIST	
add	hinzufügen, addieren
as	da, weil
bone	Knochen, Bein, Gräte (Fisch)
cardiologist, heart specialist	Kardiologe, Herzspezialist
case	Fall
consult	zu Rate ziehen, aufsuchen, konsultieren
consultant	Berater, Facharzt, Fach- (z.B. Arzt)
dermatologist, skin doctor	Dermatologe, Hautarzt
disc	Scheibe, Bandscheibe
disease	Krankheit
equipment	Ausstattung, Ausrüstung,
examine	prüfen, untersuchen
further	weiter/e, weitergehend
gall	Galle
gastro-intestinal system	Magen-Darm-Trakt
glasses	Brille
gynaecologist (UK) gynecologist (US)	Gynäkologe, Frauenarzt
imaging	Bildgebung, Abbildung, Bildwiedergabe
internal	inner/e
internist	Internist
intestines, bowels	Eingeweide
kidney	Niere
give a lecture; also: present a paper	Vortrag, Vorlesung, Referat halten
mainly	hauptsächlich
malignant	bösartig
MD	Abk. für „Medical Doctor“, Doktor der Medizin
measles	Masern
meniscus	Meniskus
nervous system	Nervensystem
oculist/ophtalmologist/eye doctor	Augenarzt

UNIT 2

EXTENDED VOCABULARY LIST	
oncologist	Onkologe, Krebsspezialist
operation	Operation, Tätigkeit, Verfahren
organ	Organ, Körperteil, Funktionseinheit
orthopaedic (UK) orthopedic (US)	orthopädisch
paediatrician/paediadrist/children's doctor	Kinderarzt
pancreas	Pankreas, Bauchspeicheldrüse
refer (to)	verweisen, überweisen, Bezug nehmen (auf)
resonance	Resonanz, Widerhall
sex	Geschlecht
skin	Haut
slip	ausrutschen, schlüpfen
spinal column/spine	Wirbelsäule
stand for	für etwas stehen, bedeuten
suffer from	leiden an/unter
throat	Kehle, Rachen, Gurgel, Hals
topic	Gesprächsgegenstand, Thema,
urinary bladder	Blase, Harnblase
urological	urologisch

Patient: Doctor, I have a serious memory problem.
I just forget everything instantly!

Doctor: So, since when have you had this problem?

Patient: What problem?

...

Doctor: Did you take those pills I gave you to improve your memory?

Patient: What pills?

(serious = ernst; memory = Gedächtnis; instantly = sofort; pills = Pillen; improve = verbessern)

3 A MEDICAL APPOINTMENT

Mrs. Kate Timberlake, a travel agent from Huddersfield (UK), is presently staying in Germany. She has got trouble with her shoulders. She decides to visit Dr. Kessler's general practice as Dr. Astrid Kessler also specializes in sports medicine. One Monday morning, Mrs. Timberlake phones to make a medical appointment. Dr. Kessler's assistant Kathrina answers the phone ...

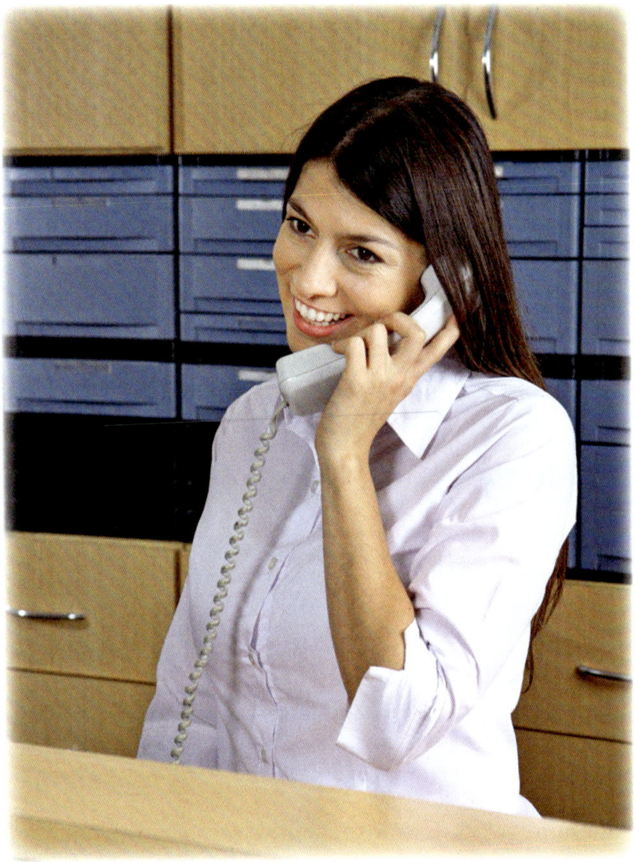

Kathrina	Praxis Dr. Kessler. Sie sprechen mit Kathrina Pohl. Guten Morgen.
Patientin	Oh, hello. This is Kate Timberlake speaking. Ah ... Do you speak English?
Kathrina	A little, yes.
Patientin	Oh, good.
Kathrina	What can I do for you?
Patientin	I'd like to book an appointment.
Kathrina	Have you been here before?

Patientin	No, I haven't.
Kathrina	What seem to be the trouble?
Patientin	I worked out at a fitness centre lately. Now, I got a sharp pain in my left shoulder and a mild pain in my right shoulder.
Kathrina	I see. Would Friday afternoon be alright for you?
Patientin	Don't you have anything earlier? Tuesday, say?
Kathrina	One moment, let me have a look ... No, I'm sorry; we have nothing free on Tuesday.
Patientin	Oh ... then, how about Wednesday afternoon?
Kathrina	Sorry, we are closed on Wednesday afternoon. Thursday is the earliest we can do. Would 8 o'clock on Thursday be OK?
Patientin	Well, 8 o'clock is a bit early.
Kathrina	Hm ... Could you come at 11.30 then?
Patientin	Yes, that's fine!
Kathrina	Right ... Could I have your name again? I didn't catch it.
Patientin	The name is T i m b e r l a k e, Mrs. Kate Timberlake.
Kathrina	Excuse me, how do you spell your surname?
Patientin	You spell it the same as the name of the famous British singer.
Kathrina	Ah, yes ... OK, Mrs. Timberlake, see you on Thursday at 11.30 then.
Patientin	Thank you very much.
Kathrina	You're welcome. Have a nice day! Bye!
Patientin	And you! Bye!

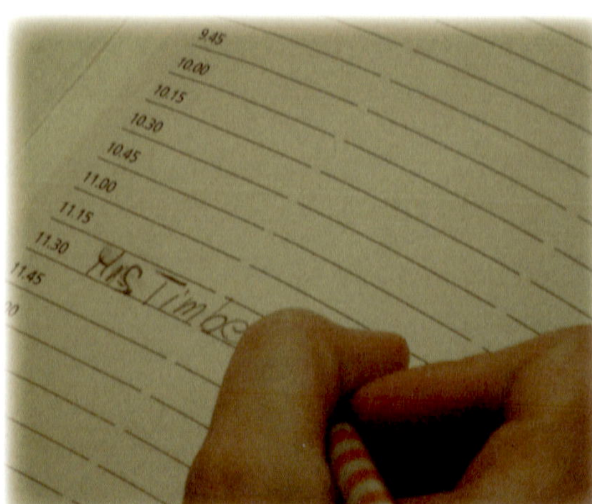

ACTIVITY 1

Find these words and expressions in the text and add them to your vocabulary list!

ein Arzttermin	Reiseverkehrskauffrau/mann	Beschwerden in der Schulter
sich entschließen	sich spezialisieren auf	Sportmedizin
Hier spricht ... (Telefon)	stechende(r) Schmerz(en)	leichte(r) Schmerz(en)
Sagen wir mal Dienstag	Wie wäre es mit ...	Wir haben geschlossen
Das passt/Das ist gut!	verstehen, fangen	buchstabieren, schreiben
Nachname (family name)	genauso wie	Bis Donnerstag!
Danke! – Gern geschehen!	Schönen Tag noch! – Tschüss!	Ebenfalls! – Tschüss!

ACTIVITY 2

Answer these questions in English!

1. Which medical field does Dr. Kessler also specialize in?
2. What is Kathrina's job?
3. Where, do you think, is she sitting at the moment?
4. Does Kathrina speak English?
5. Why is Mrs. Timberlake calling?
6. Has she visited Dr. Kessler's surgery before?
7. What medical problem has Mrs. Timberlake got?
8. Kathrina offers her an appointment on Friday. Is the day OK for Mrs. Timberlake? If not, which day would be more convenient for her?
9. Is there an appointment free on that day?
10. Wednesday afternoon is not possible. Why not?
11. What day is the earliest Kathrina can do?
12. Is it possible for Mrs. Timberlake to come on Thursday, at 8 o'clock?
13. If not, what time does Kathrina suggest?
14. Kathrina asks for Mrs. Timberlake's name again. Why?
15. What do English speaking people often reply if you say "Thank you" to them?

ACTIVITY 3

How do Kathrina and Mrs Timberlake say it in English?

1. Ich bräuchte einen Termin.
2. Würde Ihnen Freitagmorgen passen?
3. Wir haben am Dienstagnachmittag geschlossen.
4. Geht es nicht früher?
5. Könnte ich am Montag einen Termin haben?
6. Tut mir leid, wir haben am Montag nichts frei!
7. Wie wäre es mit Mittwochnachmittag?
8. Lassen Sie mich mal nachsehen.
9. Das passt!/Das ist gut!
10. Na ja, das ist ein bisschen früh!
11. Könnten Sie mir noch einmal Ihren Namen sagen?
12. Ich habe ihn nicht verstanden.
13. Ich heiße Timberlake. Mrs. Kate Timberlake.
14. Bis Dienstag!
15. Vielen Dank!
16. Gern geschehen!/Bitte!
17. Schönen Tag noch! –Tschüss!
18. Ebenfalls! – Tschüss!

UNIT 3

Patient:	Doctor, will I be able to play the piano after my hand surgery?
Surgeon:	Yes, of course!
Patient:	Great! I never could before.

(to be able to = in der Lage sein; to play the piano = Klavier spielen; hand surgery = Hand-OP, Great! = Toll!)

ACTIVITY 4

All these statements are false. Correct them. Make complete sentences!

1. Mrs. Timberlake phones to make an appointment for Friday.
2. The appointment book is full on Thursday.
3. Kathrina gives her an appointment for half past twelve.
4. Kathrina is a qualified dental employee.
5. Kathrina speaks no English at all.
6. Mrs. Timberlake is a Canadian woman who lives in Belgium.
7. Mrs. Timberlake is a tourism manager.
8. She has got the same family name as a famous British film star.
9. Mrs. Timberlake has got a walking problem.
10. Dr. Kessler does not specialize in sports medicine.

ACTIVITY 5

For Your Information

In Englisch sprechenden Ländern ist eine Zeitangabe wie z. B. 14:50 Uhr i. d. R. noch nicht so üblich wie bei uns, wird aber immer häufiger verwendet. Viele Menschen sagen dort meist noch: „2.50 p.m.“. Die Abkürzung „p.m.“ kommt aus dem Lateinischen und heißt „post meridiem“, was soviel bedeutet wie „nach Mittag“. Zeitangaben zwischen 12:01 Uhr und 24:00 Uhr werden mit dem Zusatz „p.m.“ versehen. Zeitangaben zwischen 00:01 Uhr morgens und 12:00 Uhr mittags werden mit dem Zusatz „a.m.“, d.h., „ante meridiem“, also „vor Mittag“ versehen. Beispiele: 21:45 Uhr wäre dann 9.45 p.m., oder auch 21:45 (sprich: twenty-one forty-five).

Für „zwei Uhr nachmittags“ (also volle Stunden) kann man z. B. 2 o'clock p.m. oder 14:00 hours (sprich: fourteen hundred hours) sagen. „O'clock“ sagt man nur bei vollen Stunden sowie einer 12-Stunden-Zeitrechnung! Beide Möglichkeiten, die Uhrzeit zu sagen, können nebeneinander verwendet werden, beachten Sie aber, dass vielen Briten, Iren und Nordamerikanern die 24-Stunden-Zeitrechnung noch nicht so geläufig ist.

UNIT 3

Beispiel:

Für : „Kommen Sie am 15. Januar um 13:30 Uhr“ kann man sagen:

a) Come **on** January **the** 15th, at 13.30

b) Come **on** January **the** 15th, at 1.30 p.m.

Tell the date and the time!

Do it like this: “Please, come on January the 3rd, at 16.30”

“Please, come on January the 3rd, at 4.30 p.m.”

Now, start telling the time!

03.01./12:30	24.02./08:45	10.03./16:15	17.04./09:30
30.05./14:45	09.06./11:15	31.07./18:00	13.08./12:00
19.09./08:10	10.10./11:10	11.11./11:11	24.12./20:00
06.01./21:45	02.02./23:00	18.03./10:45	20.04./14:15

ACTIVITY 6

Say it in English!

1. Kommen Sie am 23.12. um 14 Uhr.
2. Ihr Termin ist am 14.03. um 9:45 Uhr.
3. Kann ich am 02.07. um 10:30 Uhr kommen?
4. Sie bekommen einen Termin am 19.06. um 11 Uhr.
5. Ich gehe am 7. Februar um 16:15 Uhr zum Gynäkologen.
6. Am 12. Oktober um 11:45 Uhr habe ich einen Termin beim Kinderarzt.
7. Könnte ich am 04.04. um 17 Uhr kommen?
8. Bitte kommen Sie am Montag, den 13. Juli, um 16 Uhr!

ACTIVITY 7

Use the words below to make complete sentences!

1. Be/here/before?
2. I/visit/gynaecologist/next Friday.
3. I/have/appointment/dermatologists/next Tuesday.
4. Can you/come/Thursday/9:30 a.m.?
5. Can/see/doctor/June 6?
6. I/visit/oculist/last Friday.
7. My/appointment/is/Tuesday/13th/8.15 a.m.
8. Please/come/Monday/17th/9.30 a.m.
9. Is/Tuesday/October/12th/15.45/all right/with you?
10. Could/your wife/come/Wednesday/9th/4.00 p.m.?

ACTIVITY 8

Have this telephone conversation with a partner!

Assistant	Patient
1. Ihr Telefon klingelt. Sie melden sich mit dem Namen der Praxis und Ihrem eigenen Namen.	
	2. Sie grüßen und möchten gerne wissen, ob die MFA Englisch spricht.
3. Sie bejahen. Sie fragen, was Sie für die Patientin tun können.	
	4. Sie sagen, dass Sie wegen eines Schulterproblems einen Termin bräuchten. Es ist dringend. Sie haben stechende Schmerzen.

Assistant	Patient
5. Sagen Sie, dass Sie heute keine Termine mehr frei haben. Es ginge frühestens am Nachmittag des folgenden Tages.	
	6. Bitten Sie darum, am frühen Nachmittag, eventuell um 13:30 Uhr kommen zu können.
7. Fragen Sie die Patientin, ob sie auch ein wenig später kommen könnte. Um 15 Uhr sei ein Termin frei.	
	8. 15 Uhr sei für Sie auch in Ordnung.
9. Bitten Sie die Patientin, ihren Namen noch einmal zu nennen. Sie haben ihn vorhin nicht verstanden.	
	10. Wiederholen Sie Ihren Namen.
11. Bitten Sie die Patientin, ihren Namen zu buchstabieren.	
	12. Kommen Sie der Bitte nach.
13. Bestätigen Sie noch einmal den Termin der Patientin.	
	14. Sie bedanken sich.
15. Sie erwidern den Dank, wünschen einen schönen Tag und verabschieden sich.	
	16. Sie wünschen ebenfalls einen schönen Tag und verabschieden sich.

EXTENDED VOCABULARY LIST

anything	(irgend) etwas, alles, jedes Beliebige
appointment book	Terminplaner, Terminkalender
at all	überhaupt
both ... and	sowohl ... als auch
Good bye!	Auf Wiedersehen/Wiederhören!
Bye!	Tschüss!
catch	fangen, verstehen
convenient	passend, günstig
decide	(sich) entscheiden, beschließen
famous	sehr bekannt, berühmt
I'd like (to)	Ich möchte gerne
lately	kürzlich, neulich

EXTENDED VOCABULARY LIST	
look	schauen, blicken, Blick, Aussehen
mild	mild, gering
not at all	gar nicht
pain ache	Schmerz Schmerz
presently	gegenwärtig, in Kürze, zurzeit, momentan
qualified dental employee dental assistant dentist's assistant	Zahnmedizinische/r Fachangestellte/r Zahnmedizinische/r Assistent/in Zahnarzthelfer/in
qualified medical employee medical assistant doctor's assistant	Medizinische/r Fachangestellte/r Medizinische/r Assistent/in Arzthelfer/in
reply	erwidern, antworten, Antwort
sharp	stechend, scharf
spell	buchstabieren, (richtig) schreiben
suggest	vorschlagen, andeuten, hinweisen
surname (US/UK) family name (US/UK) second name (US)	Nachname
(to have) a walking problem	nicht gut Laufen können, Schwierigkeiten beim Laufen haben
to work out	hier: trainieren

Patient: Can I have an appointment on April 1?

Receptionist: The doctor can't see you before June 30.

Patient: Oh, that's too late. I might be dead by then!

Receptionist: No problem, your wife can cancel your appointment any time.

(only = hier: erst; might = könnte vielleicht; dead = tot; by then = bis dahin; cancel = absagen/stornieren; any time = jederzeit)

4 THE MENISCUS PROBLEM

Mr. Wayne Carpendile, a young professional football player from Glasgow, Scotland, is now playing for a German Second Division football club. His left knee is causing him severe problems. His physiotherapist advised him to call Dr. Astrid Kessler, who also specializes in sports medicine ...

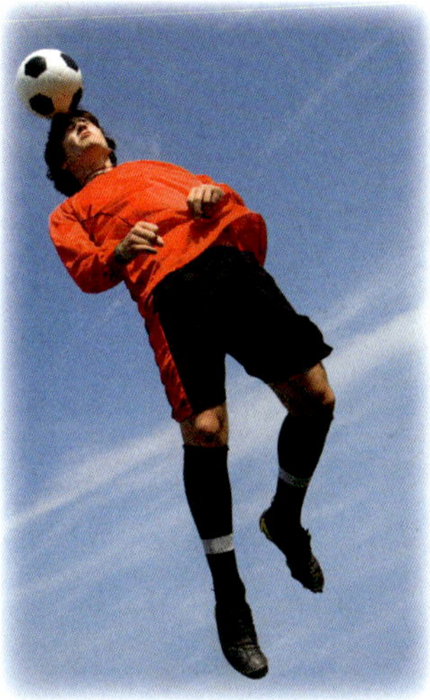

Kathrina Praxis Dr. Kessler. Sie sprechen mit Kathrina Pohl. Guten Morgen.

Patient Oh hello, this is Wayne Carpendile speaking. Could I speak to Dr. Kessler, please?

Kathrina Sorry, but that isn't possible. Dr. Kessler is busy. She's with a patient in the surgery. If you leave your number, we will call you back as soon as possible.

Patient But it's very urgent. Can't you put me through to her?

Kathrina She does not want to be disturbed while she's talking to patients. Sorry for that. Would you like to leave a message?

Patient The reason why I'm calling is my severe knee problem. It has become worse. My physiotherapist thinks it might be a meniscal tear. He advised me to see an orthopaedist or a GP specializing in sports medicine. Please tell the doctor I just cannot stand the pains anymore.

Kathrina Since when have you had this problem?

Patient Since last Saturday.

Kathrina Oh, I see ... could you hang on for a moment? I'll go and ask Dr. Kessler.

Half a minute later

Kathrina Mr. Carpendale?

Patient My name is Carpen*dile*.

Kathrina Oh, sorry. How do you spell that?

Patient (He spells it) C a r p e n d i l e.

Kathrina Yes, I got it now. Dr. Kessler told me that you can talk to her personally now. I'll put you through ...

UNIT 4

ACTIVITY 1

Find the words and expressions in the text and add them to your vocabulary list!

Zweite Bundesliga	starke Probleme	Physiotherapeut
raten, empfehlen	viel zu tun haben	Sprechzimmer
hinterlassen, zurücklassen	so bald wie möglich	dringend
durchstellen, verbinden	gestört werden	Mitteilung, Nachricht
gravierendes Knieproblem	schlimmer werden	könnte sein
Meniskusriss	etwas aushalten	warten, dranbleiben
buchstabieren, schreiben	Aha ..., Ich verstehe ...	persönlich

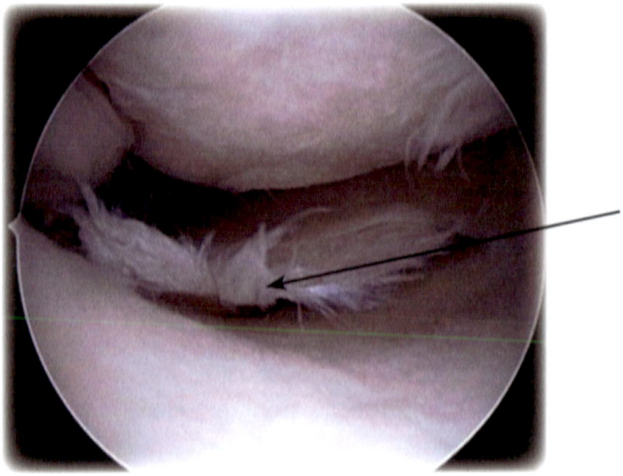

Meniscal tear

ACTIVITY 2

How would you say it in English?

1. Ich muss Frau Dr. Kessler persönlich sprechen.
2. Ich habe ein medizinisches Problem.
3. Hier spricht Wayne Carpendile.
4. Ich bin momentan beschäftigt./Ich habe im Moment viel zu tun.
5. Bitte hinterlassen Sie Ihre Nummer!
6. Es ist sehr dringend!
7. Es ist nicht möglich. Tut mir leid.
8. Frau Doktor Kessler ruft Sie so bald wie möglich zurück.
9. Dr. Kessler ist gerade im Sprechzimmer und spricht mit einem Patienten.
10 Könnten Sie mich mit ihr verbinden?
11. Sie möchte nicht gestört werden.
12. Möchten Sie eine Nachricht hinterlassen?

13. Ich habe starke Schmerzen in meinem rechten Knie.
14. Meine Schmerzen sind schlimmer geworden.
15. Ich halte sie nicht mehr aus!
16. Könnten Sie am Apparat (Telefon) bleiben?
17. Einen Moment bitte, ich stelle Sie durch/ ich verbinde Sie.

ACTIVITY 3

Answer these questions in English!

1. Who is Mr. Wayne Carpendile?
2. What is Mr. Carpendile suffering from?
3. Who sent him to Dr. Kessler?
4. Who is Dr. Kessler?
5. Why is it not possible for Mr. Carpendile to speak to Dr. Kessler personally?
6. What would Kathrina do if Wayne left his number?
7. Why is Kathrina not allowed to put patients through to Dr. Kessler?
8. What is the reason for Wayne's phone call?
9. What does Wayne's physiotherapist think it might be?
10. What happened to Wayne's knee problem?
11. How does Kathrina find out, how to write Wayne's family name?

Father: Doctor, please hurry. My son swallowed a razor-blade!
Doctor: Don't panic, I'm coming immediately. Have you done anything yet?
Father: Yes, I shaved with my electric razor instead.

(hurry = sich beeilen; swallow = verschlucken; razor-blade = Rasierklinge; to panic = in Panik geraten; immediately = gleich, sofort; yet = schon, bereits; electric razor = Elektrorasierer; instead = stattdessen)

ACTIVITY 4

All these statements are false. Correct them. Write complete sentences!

1. Mr. Carpendile is a well-known singer.
2. He has been suffering from stomach ache.
3. Dr. Kessler is a consultant neurologist.
4. Mr. Carpendile plays for a German First Division football club.
5. Mr. Carpendile has got a breathing problem.
6. His chest pains are terrible.
7. Wayne can talk to Dr. Kessler as the doctor is not busy at the moment.
8. Wayne can stand the pains easily.

UNIT 4

>>> ACTIVITY 5 >>>

Work with a partner. Ask her/him questions! Take turns!

1. Can a patient on the phone speak to the doctor in your surgery any time?
2. Are you allowed to disturb the doctor while he/she is with a patient in the consulting room/surgery?
3. Are you suffering from any pains at the moment?
4. How many consulting rooms are there in your surgery?
5. Have you ever had a knee problem?
6. If you ever had a neurological problem, what specialist would you consult?
7. Have you ever had back pains?
8. Do you know a famous professional British football player?
9. Have you ever had a headache that you could not stand anymore?
10. What would you tell a patient on the phone, if you want him or her to wait a moment?

UNIT 4

>>> ACTIVITY 6 >>>

Have this conversation with a partner!

Assistant	Patient
1. Ihr Telefon klingelt. Sie melden sich und grüßen.	
	2. Sie grüßen ebenfalls und nennen Ihren Namen. Sie möchten wissen, ob die MFA auch Englisch spricht.
3. Sie bejahen und fragen, was Sie für den Anrufer/die Anruferin tun können.	
	4. Sie bitten darum, mit dem Arzt/der Ärztin persönlich sprechen zu können.
5. Sie bedauern, dass dies nicht möglich ist, da der Arzt/die Ärztin gerade einen Patienten im Behandlungszimmer hat und nicht gestört werden möchte. Sie fragen, ob der Anrufer/die Anruferin eine Nachricht hinterlassen möchte.	
	6. Sie möchten unbedingt persönlich mit dem Arzt/der Ärztin sprechen, da Sie sehr starke Schmerzen haben, die sich verschlimmern.
7. Sie bitten den Patienten/die Patientin kurz zu warten. Sie werden den Arzt/die Ärztin fragen.	

Half a minute later

Assistant	Patient
8. Sie sagen dem Anrufer/der Anruferin, dass er/sie gleich mit dem Arzt/der Ärztin sprechen kann. Sie verbinden ...	
	9. Sie bedanken sich.
10. Sie erwidern den Dank und verabschieden sich.	

EXTENDED VOCABULARY LIST

ache, pain	Schmerz
allow	erlauben
bad/worse/worst	schlimm/schlimmer/am schlimmsten
breathing problem	Atemproblem
chest pain/back pain	Brustschmerz/Rückenschmerz
get	bekommen, verstehen, erhalten, besorgen
hang on/hold on	warten
hold the line	dranbleiben, am Telefon bleiben
leave	lassen, hinterlassen, verlassen, abfahren
personal	persönlich, privat, personenbezogen (Adjektiv)
personally	persönlich (Adverb)
profession	Beruf, Profession
reason (why)	Grund (weshalb)
refer	hier: überweisen
Second/First Division	Zweite/Erste (Bundes-)Liga
see	sehen, verstehen
severe	schlimm, schwer, stark
soon	bald
stand	aushalten, stehen, Gestell, Standplatz
stomach ache/pain	Magenschmerz(en)
urgent	dringend
well/better/best	gut/besser/am besten (Adverb)
well ...	Na ja ..., Nun gut ...

Doctor:	What seems to be the trouble?
Patient:	I've adopted a strange habit. I permanently keep talking to myself.
Doctor:	Is that so bad?
Patient:	Yes it is.
Doctor:	Why?
Patient:	I'm so boring.

(adopt = annehmen/entwickeln; strange = hier: merkwürdig, komisch; habit = Gewohnheit; permanent/ly = ständig; to keep doing something = etwas immer wieder tun; bad = schlimm; boring = langweilig)

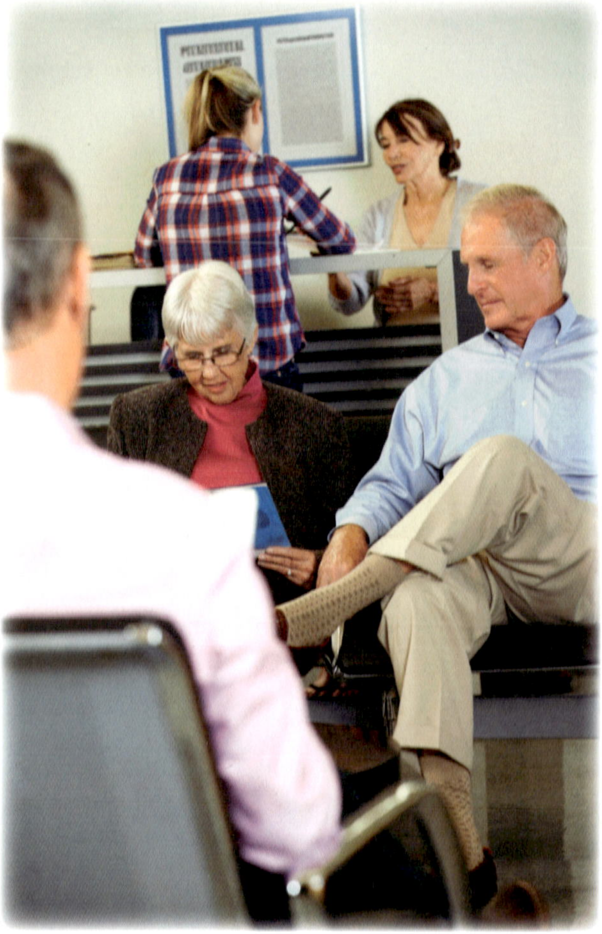

5 ASKING FOR PERSONAL DETAILS

Because of Mr. Carpendile's severe knee problem, Dr. Kessler would like to see him as soon as possible. So, Mr. Carpendile got an appointment right for the following day.

Kathrina welcomes Wayne at the reception ...

Wayne	Good morning.
Kathrina	Good Morning. How can I help you?
Wayne	My name is Carpendile, Wayne Carpendile. I talked to you on the phone yesterday. I've got an appointment with Dr. Kessler.
Kathrina	Yes, I know ... Before Dr. Kessler will see you, I need a few personal details from you.
Wayne	Sure. No problem. What would you like to know?
Kathrina	Could you please put down your Christian name, your family name and your date of birth here on this form? I also need your address here in Germany.
Wayne	Sure.
Kathrina	What is your nationality?
Wayne	I'm British.
Kathrina	OK. Could you please sign this fee agreement? I'm afraid, we must ask you to pay in cash.
Wayne	Do you also take credit cards? I've got a *Visa Card* with me.
Kathrina	Sorry. No. We don't accept credit cards but we take ***EC*** cards if you have got one.
Wayne	No problem. Do you already know how much I will have to pay?
Kathrina	Sorry, I can't tell you in advance.
Wayne	That's okay.
Kathrina	Please, take a seat in the waiting room over there. It will take a few minutes until Dr. Kessler can see you. But it won't take long.

	Ah ... I almost forgot ... May I ask you to fill in this medical history form here? It's all in English. It's very important to Dr. Kessler to know some facts about your medical history. You can complete it while you are sitting in the waiting room.
Wayne	Sure.
Britta	I'll call you in a couple of minutes ...
Wayne	Fine.

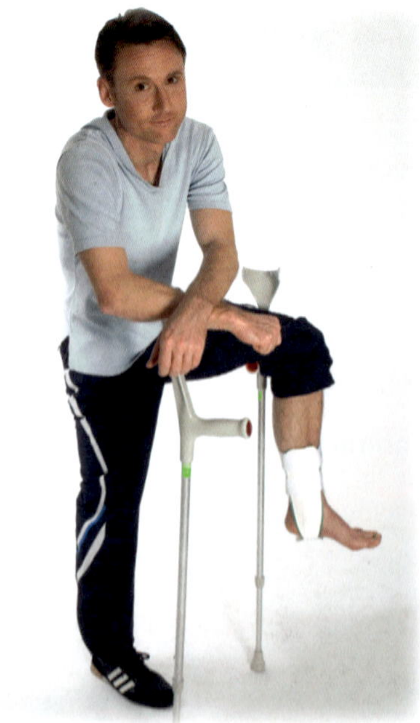

ACTIVITY 1

Find the words in the text and add them to your vocabulary list

fragen nach	persönliche Daten, Angaben	so bald wie möglich
jemanden begrüßen	ein paar	personenbezogen
hier: hinschreiben	Vorname	Nachname
Formular	Staatsangehörigkeit	unterschreiben
Honorarvereinbarung	ich fürchte ...	ich muss Sie bitten ...
(in) bar zahlen	hier: annehmen	akzeptieren, annehmen
ich kann es nicht sagen	im Voraus	Nehmen Sie Platz!
dort drüben	sich kümmern um	es dauert nicht lange
bitten	ausfüllen	Anamnesebogen
ganz auf Englisch	Einzelheiten, Tatsachen	Anamnese
während	in ein paar Minuten	Schön! Gut!

ACTIVITY 2

Can you say it in English!

1. Bitte unterschreiben Sie hier.
2. Es tut mir leid, aber wir nehmen keine Kreditkarten an.
3. Haben Sie eine EC-Karte?
4. Nehmen Sie im Wartezimmer Platz!
5. Wo ist es?/Wo befindet es sich?
6. Es ist gleich dort drüben.
7. Dr. Kessler wird Sie gleich aufrufen/Sie kommen gleich dran.
8. Darf ich Sie bitten, diesen Anamnesebogen auszufüllen?
9. Ich benötige ein paar persönliche Daten von Ihnen.
10. Nehmen Sie meine Visa Karte?
11. Tut mir leid, nein. Wir akzeptieren keine Kreditkarten.
12. Wie viel werde ich zahlen müssen?
13. Ich kann es Ihnen nicht im Voraus sagen.
14. Es wird nicht lange dauern.
15. Es dauert nur ein paar Minuten.
16. Gut!
17. Der Anamnesebogen ist ganz in Englisch geschrieben.
18. Wir benötigen einige Angaben zu Ihrer Krankengeschichte.
19. Welche Staatsangehörigkeit besitzen Sie?
20. Haben Sie einen Termin?
21. Ich benötige Ihre Adresse hier in Deutschland.
22. Könnten Sie hier bitte Ihren Vor- und Nachnamen hinschreiben?
23. Ich benötige auch Ihr Geburtsdatum.
24. Darf ich Sie bitten, bar zu zahlen?
25. Bitte unterschreiben Sie diese Honorarvereinbarung.
26. Was möchten Sie wissen?
27. Ich bin Brite.
28. Ich rufe Sie in ein paar Minuten auf.
29. Sie können das Formular ausfüllen, während Sie im Wartezimmer sitzen.

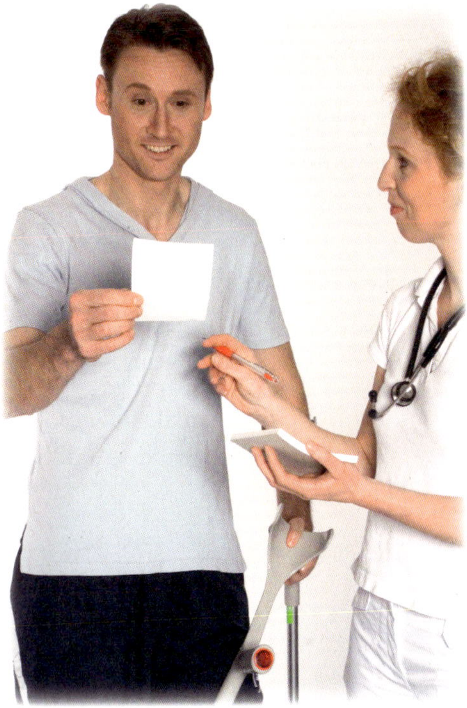

ACTIVITY 3

Please, give an answer in English! – Look at the text again.

1. What does Kathrina need from Wayne, before Dr. Kessler will see him?
2. Which personal details/data does Kathrina need from him?
3. What is Wayne's nationality?
4. Kathrina asks Wayne to sign something. What is it?
5. Kathrina only accepts two ways of payment. Which?
6. Can Wayne use his Visa card?
7. Kathrina asks Wayne to fill in a form. What form is it and why should he do it?

Patient: Doctor, it hurts when I lift my leg.

Orthopaedist: Then don't lift it!

(it hurts = es tut weh; to lift = heben,anheben)

ACTIVITY 4

Work with a partner. Ask her/him questions!

1. What is your nationality?
2. Have you ever filled in a medical history form?
3. Has any doctor ever asked about your medical history?
4. Do you take credit cards in/at your surgery?
5. You want a patient to sit down in the waiting room. How would you politely tell him to do this?

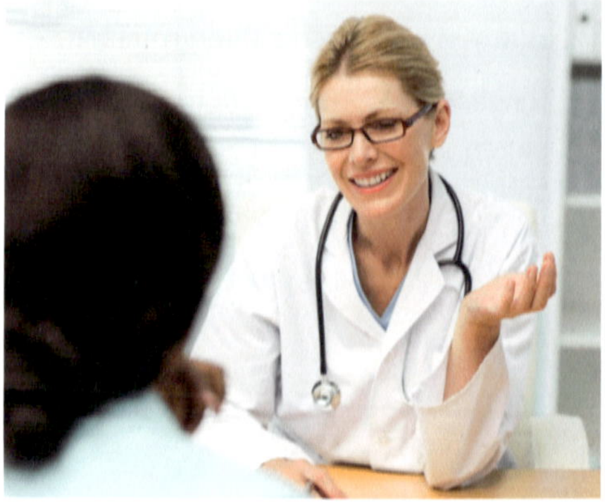

ACTIVITY 5

Have this conversation with a partner in English!

Patient	Assistant
1. Sie betreten die Praxis und gehen zur Anmeldung. Sie möchten wissen, ob in dieser Praxis jemand Englisch spricht.	
	2. Sie bejahen und fragen, was Sie für den Patienten/die Patientin tun können.
3. Sie stellen sich vor und fragen, ob Sie heute noch einen Termin haben könnten.	
	4. Sie bejahen, sagen aber, dass es lange dauern kann.
5. Sie erwidern, dass dies kein Problem sei. Sie haben genügend Zeit.	
	6. Sie legen dem Patienten/der Patientin ein Formular vor und bitten ihn/sie, darin patientenbezogene Angaben zu machen (Vor- und Nachname, Geburtsdatum, Adresse). Erkundigen Sie sich auch nach seiner/ihrer Staatsangehörigkeit.
7. Sie geben die gewünschten Auskünfte.	
	8. Weisen Sie den Patienten/die Patientin darauf hin, dass Sie nur Barzahlung oder Zahlung mit EC-Karte akzeptieren können.
9. Sagen Sie, dass das kein Problem sei.	
	10. Bitten Sie ihn/sie auch, eine Honorarvereinbarung zu unterschreiben. Anschließend bitten Sie ihn/sie, Angaben zu seiner/ihrer Anamnese zu machen. Sagen Sie dem Patienten/der Patientin, weshalb Angaben zur Krankengeschichte für den Arzt wichtig sind. Geben Sie dem Patienten/der Patientin einen Stift und weisen Sie ihn darauf hin, dass er die Formulare und den Anamnesebogen gerne im Wartezimmer ausfüllen kann.
11. Sie wissen nicht, wo das Wartezimmer ist und erkundigen sich, wo es sich befindet.	
	12. Sie sagen, dass es sich gleich gegenüber befindet.

EXTENDED VOCABULARY LIST	
address	Adresse, Anschrift
advance/in advance	voraus/im Voraus
afraid (of)	Angst haben (vor), leider
cash	(in) bar, Bargeld, Barzahlung,
Christian name (brit)/first name (US)	Vorname
couple (of)	einige, ein paar
fact	Tatsachen, Einzelheiten
fee	Gebühr, Entgelt, Honorar
fee agreement	Honorarvereinbarung
fill in	ausfüllen
form	Formular, Form, Umgangsform
means of payment	Zahlungsmittel
medical history	Anamnese, medizinische Vorgeschichte
nationality	Nationalität, Staatsangehörigkeit
personal details	persönliche Angaben, personenbezogene Angaben
polite/ly	höflich
previous	vorherig, vorhergehend
put down	niederschreiben, herabsetzen
right opposite	gleich gegenüber
seat	Sitz, Sitzgelegenheit, Platz,
see to	sich kümmern um, nach etwas sehen
sign	unterschreiben, unterzeichnen, Zeichen
Sure!	Sicher! Na klar!
Take	annehmen, nehmen, ertragen

Orthopaedist: Did you know that there are more than 1000 bones in the human body?

Patient: Shhh, doctor! My dog is outside in the waiting room.

(Shhh! = Pssst!; bones = Knochen; human body = menschlicher Körper)

6 AN ACCIDENT AT WORK

Mr. Francis Fulton is a construction worker from Ireland. He is employed by a local German building company. The company has got a construction site near the surgery of the general practitioner Dr. Astrid Kessler. Mr. Fulton had bad luck at work. He slipped and fell over an iron bar lying on the ground. His left arm is badly bruised and he cannot move it anymore. One of his workmates called the surgery and wanted to know if anyone speaks English there, because Mr. Fulton's German is poor. His workmate took him to the surgery. Dr. Kessler's assistant Kathrina is sitting at reception ...

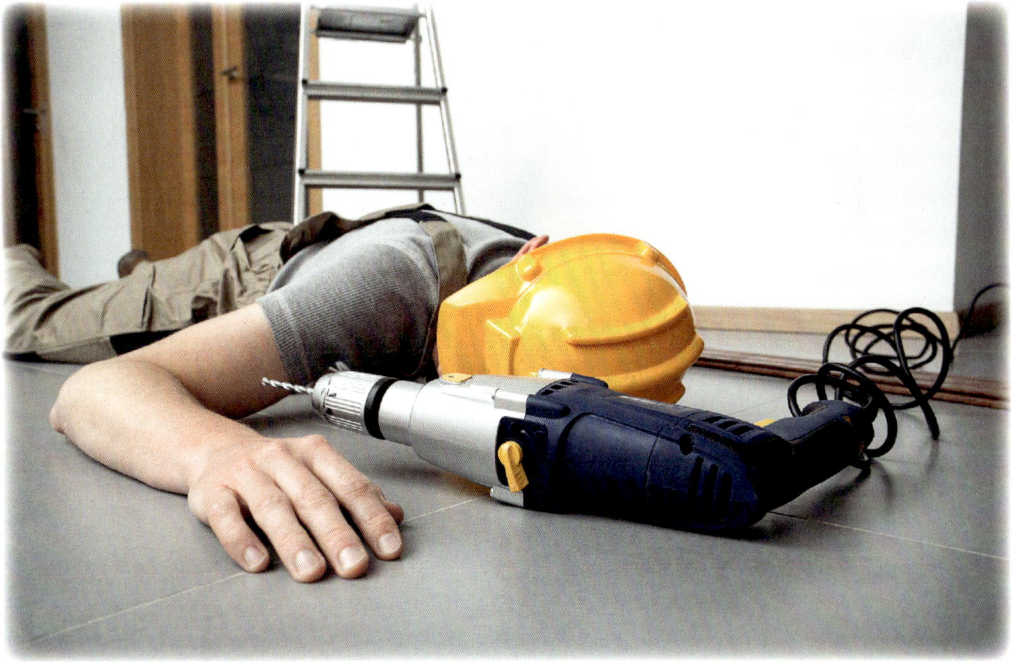

Workmate Guten Morgen. Ich habe vorhin bei Ihnen angerufen. Mein irischer Kollege hatte einen Unfall auf unserer Baustelle. Außerdem spricht er kaum Deutsch.

Kathrina Kein Problem. Setzen Sie ihn in den Behandlungsraum. Ich komme gleich.

Kathrina comes in

Mr. Fulton Hello. My name is Fulton. Francis Fulton.

Kathrina Hello, Mr. Fulton, it seems you had an accident at work?

Mr. Fulton Yes.

Kathrina Before Dr. Kessler will see you, I need to know the name of your company's "Berufsgenossenschaft".

Mr. Fulton "Berufsgenossenschaft"? What's that?

Kathrina That's your employer's accident insurance. It covers medical expenses for the treatment of accidents which happened at work.

Mr. Fulton I see. My boss gave me this note here. He said that there's everything you need to know written on it.

Kathrina OK, thanks. Do you have medical insurance?

Mr. Fulton Look, I have this medical card here ...

Kathrina Fine. I only need to know the name of your health insurance company but I don't need your medical card if you had an accident at work.
Well, then I need your date of birth, your employer's name and address and your telephone number at work.

Mr. Fulton (He gives her all the details ...)

Kathrina What's your occupation?

Mr. Fulton I'm a construction worker.

Kathrina How long have you been a construction worker?

Mr. Fulton For 15 years now.

Kathrina Good. Has the accident happened today?

Mr. Fulton Yes. Half an hour ago, at about 9.30 a.m.

Kathrina What is your nationality?

Mr. Fulton I'm Irish.

Kathrina When did you start work and what time would you have stopped work today?

Mr. Fulton I started at 7.30 this morning and we usually stop work at 4 o'clock p.m.

Kathrina How did the accident happen?

Mr. Fulton (He tells her how it happened)

Kathrina The doctor will see you in a couple of minutes

15 minutes later, after the examination by Dr. Kessler

Kathrina Well, Mr Fulton, Dr. Kessler thinks it might be a fracture.
We will have to send you to a "Durchgangsarzt".

Mr. Fulton Who is that?

Kathrina That's a specialist for accident injuries. He also is an accident insurance consultant treating injuries of employees who had an accident at work.
His address is on this form. Your colleague can take you there by car. I'll call their surgery to tell them that you are coming ...

ACTIVITY 1

Find the following words in the text and add them to your vocabulary list

Arbeitsunfall	ein Monteur, ein Bauarbeiter	er ist beschäftigt bei
ortsansässig, lokal	Bauunternehmer	eine Baustelle
Pech haben	während der Arbeit	er rutschte aus
eine Eisenstange	auf dem Boden liegend	ein Bruch
schwer gequetscht	Arbeitskollege, Kumpel	schlechtes Deutsch
in die Praxis bringen	Anmeldung	Arbeitgeber
Unfallversicherung	Ausgaben für medizinische Behandlung decken	Notizzettel
Krankenversicherung	KV-Karte	Arbeitgeber
Geburtsdatum	Beruf, Berufstätigkeit	Staatsangehörigkeit
die Arbeit beginnen	die Arbeit beenden	in ein paar Minuten
Fraktur	Unfallarzt (Spezialist für unfallbedingte Verletzungen)	im Auftrag einer BG tätiger Unfallarzt (Durchgangsarzt)

ACTIVITY 2

Answer these questions in English!

1. Where did the accident in the text happen?
2. What is Mr. Fulton's occupation?
3. Where is the construction site located?
4. Mr. Fulton had bad luck. What happened to him?
5. Is lifting his left arm a problem to him at the moment?
6. Which trouble has he got?
7. Who took him to the surgery?
8. Which are the first two things Kathrina asks him about?

9. Has he got a medical card?
10. Which additional personal details does Katharina need?
11. Which additional personal details does Kathrina need?
12. For how many years has Mr. Fulton been a construction worker?
13. Mr. Fulton cannot move his left arm. What does Dr. Kessler think about this problem?
14. Where will Dr. Kessler send him for further treatment?
15. What is a "Durchgangsarzt"? Explain!
16. How does Mr. Fulton get to the accident insurance consultant?

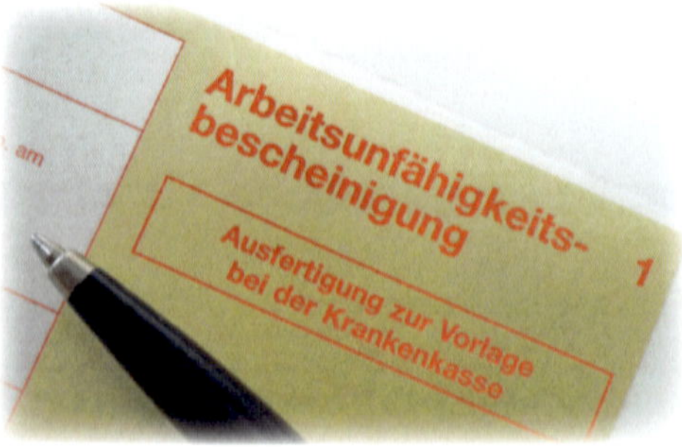

ACTIVITY 3

Can you say it in English?

1. Seine Firma hat eine Baustelle in der Nähe der Praxis.
2. Er ist bei einer ortsansässigen Baufirma beschäftigt.
3. Er rutschte aus.
4. Er fiel über eine Eisenstange.
5. Die Eisenstange lag auf dem Boden.
6. Er kann seinen linken Arm nicht mehr bewegen.
7. Es könnte eine Fraktur sein.
8. Den Arm zu heben ist für ihn ein Problem.
9. Einer seiner Kollegen rief die Praxis an.
10. Sein Deutsch ist schlecht.
11. Können Sie ihn in die Praxis bringen?
12. Er hatte einen Arbeitsunfall.
13. Wenn Sie einen Arbeitsunfall hatten, benötige ich keine KV-Karte.
14. Könnte ich die Anschrift Ihres Arbeitgebers haben?
15. Was machen Sie beruflich?
16. Wie heißt die Berufsgenossenschaft Ihres Arbeitgebers?
17. Ist der Unfall heute passiert?
18. Welche Staatsangehörigkeit besitzen Sie?
19. Wann begannen Sie heute Morgen mit der Arbeit?
20. Wann werden Sie heute Ihre Arbeit beenden?
21. Könnten Sie mir schildern, wie der Unfall passiert ist?
22. Wir schicken Sie zu einem Durchgangsarzt.
23. Seine Anschrift finden Sie auf diesem Formular.
24. Könnten Sie Ihren Kollegen fragen, ob er Sie mit dem Wagen hinbringen kann?
25. Ich rufe die Praxis dort an, und teile ihnen mit, dass Sie kommen.

A man ran into a doctor's office.
"Doctor!" The man screamed, "I've lost my memory!"
"When did this happen?" asked the doctor.
The man looked at him and said, "When did what happen?"

(scream = schreien; to lose the memory = das Gedächtnis verlieren)

ACTIVITY 4

Ask your partner questions! Take turns!

1. What would you do if a patient, who had an accident and cannot walk without help, enters your surgery?
2. A patient, who had an accident at work, enters your surgery. What questions would you ask him?
3. Would you ask for a medical card, if a patient had an accident at work?
4. What is your occupation?
5. Who is a "Durchgangsarzt"?

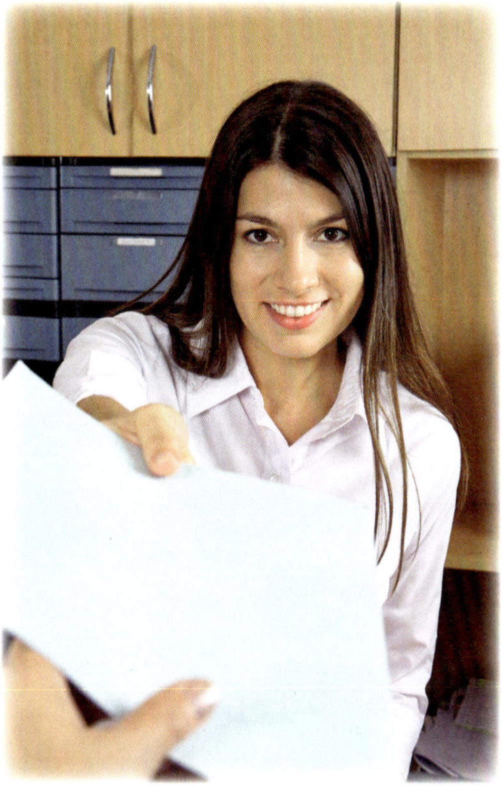

ACTIVITY 5

An English speaking patient had an accident at work.
Have this conversation with him/her!

Assistant	Patient
1. Fragen Sie, ob er/sie einen Unfall hatte.	
	2. Erklären Sie, dass es sich um einen Arbeitsunfall handelt.
3. Fragen Sie, welche Verletzungen er/sie sich zugezogen hat und wo es schmerzt.	
	4. Geben Sie Auskunft über Ihre Verletzung(en) und Schmerzen.
5. Sagen Sie dem Patienten/der Patientin, dass sich der Arzt gleich darum kümmern wird.	
	6. Erwidern Sie etwas.
7. Fragen Sie den Patienten/die Patientin nach seiner Krankenkasse und nach der der Berufsgenossenschaft seines Arbeitgebers.	
	8. Geben Sie die gewünschten Auskünfte. Fragen Sie, ob Sie ihre KV-karte benötigen.
9. Sagen Sie, dass Sie im Falle eines Arbeitsunfalls keine KV-Karte benötigen	
	10. Erwidern Sie etwas darauf.
11. Fragen Sie den Patienten/die Patientin nun nach seinem/ihrem Namen, Geburtsdatum, Adresse hier in Deutschland, Heimatadresse, Namen und Telefonnummer des Arbeitgebers und seinem/ihrem Beruf.	
	12. Geben Sie die gewünschten Auskünfte.
13. Fragen Sie, seit wann er/sie seinen/ihren Beruf bereits ausübt.	
	14. Geben Sie darüber Auskunft.
15. Fragen Sie nach seiner/ihrer Staatsangehörigkeit.	
	16. Geben Sie darüber Auskunft.
17. Fragen Sie, wann genau der Unfall geschah (Tag/Uhrzeit).	
	18. Geben Sie darüber Auskunft.

Assistant	Patient
19. Bitten Sie den Patienten/die Patientin um eine genaue Schilderung des Unfallhergangs.	
	20. Schildern Sie den Unfall.
21. Sagen Sie dem Patienten/der Patientin, dass Sie ihn/sie nach der Untersuchung zu einem Durchgangsarzt schicken werden.	
	22. Sie möchten gerne wissen, was ein „Durchgangsarzt“ ist.
23. Erklären Sie es.	
	24. Fragen Sie, wie Sie hinkommen. Sie können kaum laufen.
25. Schlagen Sie dem Patienten/der Patientin vor, einen Arbeitskollegen zu bitten, ihn/sie hinzubringen. Falls dies nicht möglich ist, könnte man auch einen Krankenwagen anfordern.	

Patient: My wife beats me, doctor!

Doctor: Oh dear! How often?

Patient: Every time we play chess!

(beat = schlagen; Oh dear! = Du lieber Himmel!; every time = jedes Mal; chess = Schach)

EXTENDED VOCABULARY LIST	
arm	Arm
bad luck	Missgeschick, Pech, Unglück
bar	Stange, Balken
charge, fee	Gebühr
employ	beschäftigen
employee	Arbeitnehmer

EXTENDED VOCABULARY LIST	
employer	Arbeitgeber
good luck	Glück
hurt **Does it hurt?**	schmerzen Schmerzt es? Tut es weh?
injured	verletzt
injury **accident injury**	Verletzung unfallbedingte Verletzung
lay down/lay back	hinlegen (Sache)/zurücklehnen
lie, **lying**	liegen, lügen liegend, lügend
lie down	hinlegen (Person)
(be) located	liegen, sich befinden
location	Standort, Lage, Position
(be) lucky	Glück haben
medical card	KV-Karte, Chipkarte
note	Notizzettel
occupation	Beruf
poor	arm, schlecht, armselig
specialist for accident injuries	Unfallarzt
(be) unlucky	Pech haben

Patient: Doctor, are you sure I'm suffering from cancer? I've once heard about a doctor treating someone suffering from cancer and finally he died of typhus.

Doctor: Don't worry, this won't happen to me. If I treat someone suffering from cancer he **will die** of cancer.

(be sure = sich sicher sein; to suffer from = leiden an; cancer = Krebs; to have once heard about someone = früher einmal von jem. gehört haben; to treat with = behandeln wegen; finally = schließlich; to die of = sterben an)

7 A TALK ABOUT SYMPTOMS

Mrs. Karen Brady and her husband have rented an apartment right upstairs from Dr. Kessler's general practice. Karen and her husband Michael do not speak German yet. Now, Mrs. Brady has been feeling ill for a while. It is late afternoon. Her husband is meeting Kathrina outside the surgery ...

Mr. Brady Hi, Kathrina.

Kathrina Hi, Mr. Brady. How's your wife today?

Mr. Brady Not great, I'm afraid. She's still feeling tired and doesn't seem to have much energy. She's got a stiff neck, a sore throat and is feeling feverish. Her bones are aching and she's got a terrible headache. I guess she's caught a bad cold.

Kathrina Has she got a temperature?

Mr. Brady I guess so.

Kathrina Have you been in a forest, in a garden or in a meadow lately?

Mr. Brady Ah ... yes ... about three weeks ago we plucked flowers with the kids in a meadow. Why do you want to know?

Kathrina Well, it might also have been a tick bite. You should know that some ticks in Germany can communicate meningoencephalitis or borreliosis. Flu-like symptoms are typical if you are infected.

Mr. Brady Oh, is that dangerous?

Kathrina Yes, I'm afraid it is. But we should not assume the worst. A higher body temperature can be normal. Those symptoms could mean a lot of things. It could even just be flu. Your wife should see Dr. Kessler and have a blood specimen taken. Just to make sure.

Mr. Brady I guess you're right. She should see a doctor. I'm very worried, you know.

Kathrina Good. But I'm sure, there's nothing to worry about.

Mr. Brady That's nice of you to say. Let's see what Dr. Kessler says.

Kathrina Tell your wife to see Dr. Kessler any time tomorrow!

Mr. Brady Shall I book an appointment for her?

Kathrina That won't be necessary. We won't be very busy tomorrow.

ACTIVITY 1

Find these words and expressions and add them to your vocabulary list!

ein Gespräch über	Symptome	verheiratet
mieten	Mietwohnung (US)	direkt über, direkt darüber
Nicht (gerade) gut, fürchte ich	scheinen	viel Energie
steifer Hals/Nacken	Halsschmerzen	sich fiebrig fühlen
die Knochen	es tut weh, es schmerzt	Kopfschmerzen
ich vermute, ich nehme an	Erkältung	sich eine Erkältung zuziehen/holen
Fieber	Wald, Forst	Wiese
kürzlich, in letzter Zeit	vor drei Wochen	Blumen pflücken
ein Zeckenbiss	eine Krankheit übertragen	grippeähnlich
typisch	infiziert, angesteckt	Meningoenzephalitis
schädlich, gefährlich	annehmen	das Schlimmste
erhöhte Körpertemperatur	bedeuten	vieles
sogar	es ist nur, lediglich	die Grippe (Influenza)
Blutprobe (ent)nehmen	um sicher zu gehen	beunruhigt sein
jederzeit	notwendig, nötig	hier: voll sein

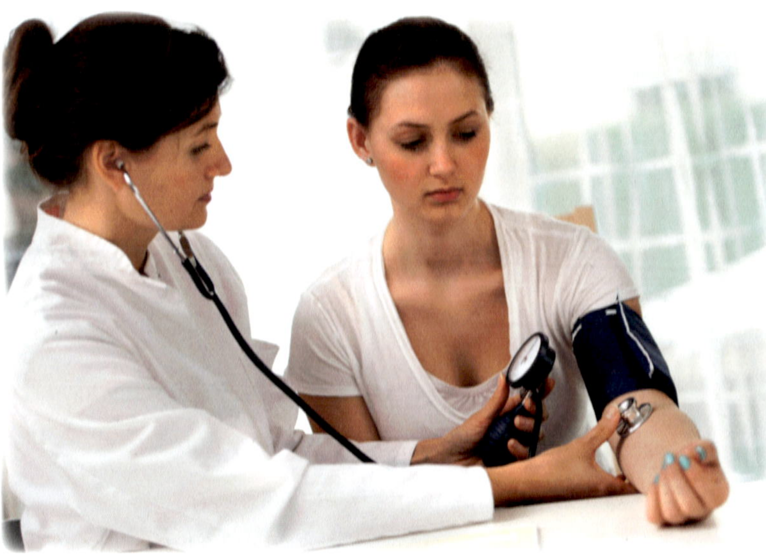

ACTIVITY 2

Answer the questions in English!

1. How has Mrs. Brady been feeling?
2. What about her energy?
3. Which symptoms is she suffering from?
4. What does Mrs. Brady's husband assume?
5. What does Kathrina want to know?
6. What did the Bradys do about three weeks ago?
7. What does Kathrina assume?
8. Are all the ticks in Germany harmless?
9. What does Kathrina say to calm down/ to reassure Mr. Brady?
10. What does she advise Mrs. Brady to do as soon as possible?

ACTIVITY 3

Can you say it in English!

1. Ich fühle mich die ganze Zeit (schon) krank/unwohl.
2. Hallo Kathrina. Wie geht's dir?
3. Na ja, nicht so toll, fürchte ich.
4. Ich fühle mich immer noch müde und habe nicht viel Energie
5. Hast du Halsschmerzen?
6. Ich habe einen (ganz) steifen Nacken.
7. Ich fühle mich fiebrig.
8. Ich glaube, ich habe mir eine Erkältung eingefangen.
9. Alle meine Knochen tun mir weh/ schmerzen.
10. Hast du auch Kopfschmerzen?
11. Ich denke nicht, dass es nur eine harmlose Erkältung ist.
12. Hast du Fieber?
13. Ich glaube schon.
14. Es könnte auch ein Zeckenbiss gewesen sein.
15. Manche Zecken übertragen Meningoenzephalitis oder Borreliose.
16. Diese Krankheiten sind sehr gefährlich.
17. Wir sollten aber nicht (gleich) das Schlimmste annehmen.
18. Eine erhöhte Körpertemperatur kann normal sein.
19. Die Symptome könnten Vieles bedeuten.
20. Ich bin (mir) sicher, es ist nichts weswegen man sich sorgen müsste.

ACTIVITY 4

Have this conversation with a partner!

You	Partner
1. Begrüßen Sie Ihre Freundin und fragen Sie, wie es ihrer Mutter geht.	
	2. Erzählen Sie ihr, dass es Ihrer Mutter nicht so gut geht. Wahrscheinlich hat sie sich eine schlimme Erkältung zugezogen.
3. Fragen Sie, wie sie sich momentan fühlt und welche Symptome aufgetreten sind.	
	4. Erzählen Sie, was sie alles hat: (schreckliche Kopfschmerzen, Nackensteife, Halsschmerzen, mangelnde Energie, Müdigkeit, Knochenschmerzen).
5. Erkundigen Sie sich, ob sie auch eine erhöhte Körpertemperatur hat.	
	6. Sagen Sie, dass Sie das vermuten, weil sie sich fiebrig fühlt.
7. Äußern Sie die Vermutung, dass es sich auch um einen Zeckenbiss handeln könnte. Manche Zecken können Meningoenzephalitis oder Borreliose verursachen. Grippeähnliche Symptome sind typisch für eine Infektion.	
	8. Äußern Sie, dass Sie sich jetzt große Sorgen machen.
9. Beruhigen Sie die Freundin und weisen Sie darauf hin, dass diese Symptome alle möglichen Ursachen haben könnten. Es könnte sich auch um eine Grippe handeln.	
	10. Sagen Sie der Freundin, dass Ihre Mutter für morgen bereits einen Termin beim Allgemeinarzt hat.
11. Raten Sie der Freundin, dass ihre Mutter auch eine Blutuntersuchung durchführen lassen sollte – nur um sicherzugehen. Betonen Sie nochmals, dass Sie davon überzeugt sind, dass es nichts ist, weswegen man sich Sorgen machen müsse.	
	12. Bedanken Sie sich für die beruhigenden Worte Ihrer Freundin.

Back to our story...

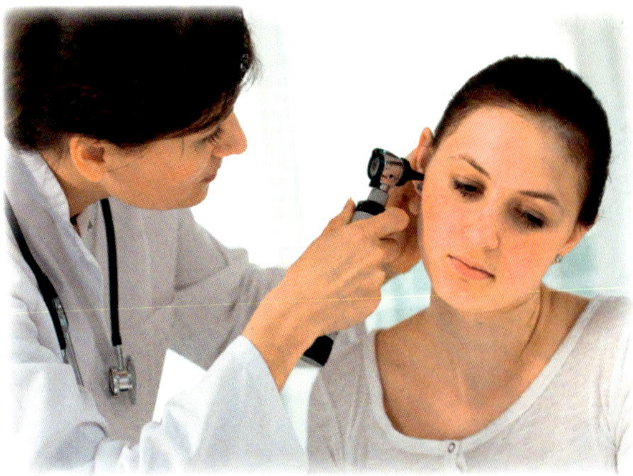

The symptoms have grown worse. Now, Mrs. Brady has even got chest pains and her entire lower body, mainly the area around the stomach, the bowels and the kidneys have become very sensitive. As she will have to stand the pains until the next day, she thinks of taking a strong pain-killer. So, in the early evening she starts taking painkilling tablets. In one of the drawers in her kitchen Karen Brady found half a box of paracetamol tablets. Paracetamol is a very efficient analgesic.

Next day, at 8.15 a.m., Mrs. Brady enters Dr. Kessler's general practice ...

Kathrina Good morning, Mrs. Brady.

Mrs. Brady Good morning, Kathrina.

Kathrina Oh, you're looking rather ill, Mrs. Brady ...

Mrs. Brady Yes, every part of my body seems to be aching. I already took almost half a box of paracetamol tablets. But they don't seem to relieve the pains at all ...

Kathrina Well, I understand that you took an analgesic for your pains already. But we should find out what exactly the causes of all these symptoms are. You know, self-medication, that is taking any tablets without an exact diagnosis, can be dangerous. OK, you can go to room 2 straight away. My colleague Eva will be with you in a minute.

In the examining room

Eva OK, let's take your body temperature. Hm ... thirty-nine point five (39,5° degrees centigrade). Seems, you got a temperature! That's why you are looking so feverish. Then, let's measure your blood pressure ... I'm afraid, your blood pressure is strikingly increased. It's hundred and sixty over over ninety-five (160/95)

Mrs. Brady Yes, I know. I also suffer from high blood pressure ...

ACTIVITY 5

Say it in English!

1. Die Symptome werden (langsam) schlimmer.
2. Ich habe Brustschmerzen.
3. Mein ganzer Körper tut weh.
4. Alles ist sehr schmerzempfindlich geworden.
5. Der Magen, der Darm und die Nieren schmerzen.
6. Ich kann die Schmerzen nicht mehr aushalten.
7. Ich habe ein starkes Schmerzmittel genommen.
8. Ich habe damit begonnen, schmerzstillende Tabletten einzunehmen.
9. In einer meiner Schubladen fand ich eine Packung Schmerztabletten.
10. Ich nahm eine halbe Packung Paracetamol.
11. Es ist ein sehr wirksames Analgetikum.
12. Sie sehen ziemlich krank aus.
13. Die Schmerztabletten haben meine Schmerzen überhaupt nicht erleichtert.
14. Was ist die Ursache für all meine Schmerzen?
15. Ohne eine genaue Diagnose irgendwelche Tabletten einzunehmen, ist sehr gefährlich.
16. Man sollte immer zuerst einen Arzt aufsuchen, bevor man irgendwelche Tabletten einnimmt.
17. Der Arzt wird dann die wirksamste Medikation verschreiben.
18. Der Arzt wird dies tun, wenn er alle Untersuchungsbefunde hat.
19. Selbstmedikation kann gefährlich sein!
20. Mein Blutdruck ist 120/80. Das ist normal.

ACTIVITY 6

Ask your partner questions! Take turns!

1. Do you think that paracetamol would relieve headache?
2. How often do you take painkilling tablets?
3. Do you think that it could be dangerous to take medicines without having seen a doctor before?
4. Am I looking ill?
5. What is the best way to relieve headache?
6. How can you catch meningoencephalitis?
7. If I caught a really bad flu. What would you advise me to do?
8. Is a "cold" the same as "flu"?
9. What word would many English or American people use if they had a fever?
10. What should you not forget to do after you have been lying in the grass?

EXTENDED VOCABULARY LIST	
advise	raten, beraten
analgesic	schmerzstillend, Analgetikum, Schmerzmittel
apartment (US); flat (Brit.)	Mietwohnung
area	Gegend, Gebiet
assume	annehmen, vermuten
blood test	Blutuntersuchung
bowel movement	Stuhlgang
bowels	Eingeweide
box	Schachtel, Behälter
calm down	(sich) beruhigen
catch	fangen, sich einfangen (Krankheit), verstehen
cause	Ursache, Grund, verursachen
centigrade/celsius	Celsius Grade
chest	Brust, Brustkorb, Kiste
chest pains	Brustschmerzen
cold	kalt, Kälte, Erkältung
communicate	kommunizieren, übertragen (Krankheit)
degrees	Grad, Grade
draw	ziehen, malen, zeichnen
drawer	Schublade
drug	Medikament, Arzneimittel, Droge, Rauschgift
effective	effektiv, wirkungsvoll, tatsächlich
efficient	wirksam, effizient, tüchtig
entire	ganz, gänzlich, vollständig, total, uneingeschränkt
even	sogar
feeling ill	unwohl, (sich) krank fühlen
fever, temperature	Fieber
flu	Grippe

EXTENDED VOCABULARY LIST	
flu-like	grippeähnlich
forest	Wald, Forst
Great!	Toll! Super!
grow	wachsen, langsam zunehmen
guess	annehmen, raten, vermuten, Vermutung, Schätzung
harmful	schädlich, nachteilig
harmless	unschädlich, harmlos, ungefährlich
increase	zunehmen, Zunahme
late	spät
lately	kürzlich, neulich
lawn	Rasen
married to	verheiratet mit
meadow	Wiese
mean	bedeuten, meinen, beabsichtigen, gemein, schäbig
measure	messen, Maß, Maßeinheit
medication	Medikation, Medikamente, medizinische Behandlung
medicine	Arznei, Medizin, Heilkunde, Medikament
neck	Hals, Genick
Not great!	Nicht so toll!
outside	außerhalb, außer Haus
pluck	pflücken
proper	ordentlich, passend, geeignet, angemessen, ordnungsgemäß, höflich
reading	hier: der (abgelesene) Wert
reassure	beruhigen, zusichern, Gefühl der Sicherheit geben
relief	Erleichterung, Entlastung
relieve	erleichtern, befreien, Erleichterung

EXTENDED VOCABULARY LIST	
(to) report sick **(to) call in sick**	sich krank melden
seem	Anschein, scheinen, wirken
sensible	vernünftig
sensitive	empfindlich, sensibel, spürbar
sore	entzündet, wund, schmerzhaft, beleidigt, empfindlich
sore throat	Halsentzündung, Halsschmerzen
strikingly increased	deutlich erhöht
temperature, fever	Temperatur, Fieber
tick bite	Zeckenbiss
upstairs from	oberhalb von (innerhalb eines Gebäudes)
(for a) while	eine Zeit lang

A black African man opened the door to a doctor's waiting room and walked straight to the door of the consulting room on the other side. He ignored all the patients waiting there. As he was about to open the door of the doctor's surgery, a woman jumped up and caught him by his arm. "No, we come before you" she said.

The black man answered in the same tone: "No, you come after me – I'm the doctor"

(straight = geradewegs; consulting room = Sprechzimmer; ignore = ignorieren; to be about to = im Begriff sein zu; jump up = aufspringen; catch = hier: packen; tone = Tonfall; surgery = hier: Behandlungsraum)

UNIT 7

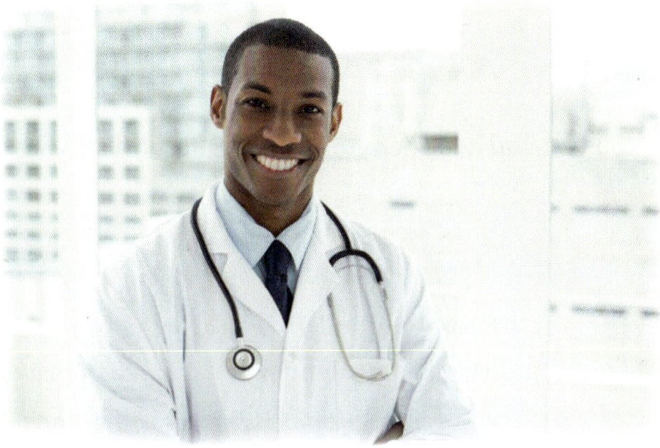

8 DEALING WITH BREAST CANCER

Qualified medical employees of a German vocational college are asked to draw up a flyer aimed for English speaking female patients of consultant gynaecologists. Please, read what they wrote:

Dear patient,

We are sure, that you are already aware of the dangers of breast cancer. You will certainly know that clinical examinations once in a while are **not enough** to diagnose breast cancer. Examine your breasts regularly! Do it once a month! This is especially important if there is a history of cancer in your family. If you find a lump in your breast, please see your gynaecologist as soon as possible to find out what the lump is. The lump can just be a harmless cyst, but it might also be a benign or even a malignant tumour. To make sure, we will do further examinations and tests to find out more. Please, do not hesitate to ask our experienced staff if you have any questions. Our assistants will give you any information you need.

ACTIVITY 1

Find these words in the text and add them to your vocabulary list!

umgehen mit	Brustkrebs, Mammakarzinom	Berufsschule
bitten	entwerfen (Schriftstück)	Handzettel, Faltblatt, Flyer
Englisch sprechend	weibliche Patienten	sich bewusst sein
sicher, sicherlich	klinische Untersuchung	hin und wieder

prüfen, untersuchen	regelmäßig	einmal pro Monat
besonders wichtig	Vorgeschichte (klinisch)	Knoten, Geschwulst
harmlose Zyste	gutartig, benigne	maligne, bösartige Geschwulst
sicher gehen	weitere Tests/ Untersuchungen	zögern
erfahren, sachkundig	Personal, Mitarbeiter	irgendwelche Fragen
Helfer/innen	jede (z.B.) Information	Information/en

ACTIVITY 2

Bitte übersetzen Sie einer nicht Englisch sprechenden Patientin den Inhalt des Handzettels!

ACTIVITY 3

Can you say it in English!

1. Entwerfen Sie bitte einen Hand-zettel für das Wartezimmer!
2. Für welche Patienten ist er be-stimmt?
3. Wir sind uns der Gefahren bereits bewusst.
4. Sie werden das sicher bereits wissen.
5. Eine sporadische klinische Untersuchung der Brust reicht nicht aus.
6. Sie sollten Ihre Brust regelmäßig abtasten/untersuchen.
7. Ist in Ihrer Familie bereits Brustkrebs vorgekommen?
8. Ich habe einen Knoten in meiner linken Brust gefunden.
9. Ich werde mir so bald wie möglich einen Termin geben lassen.
10. Der Knoten könnte aber auch nur eine harmlose Zyste sein.
11. Zögern Sie nicht, Ihren Gynäkologen zu fragen.
12. Unser Praxispersonal ist sehr routiniert/erfahren.
13. Unser Praxispersonal wird Ihnen jede Auskunft geben, die Sie benötigen.

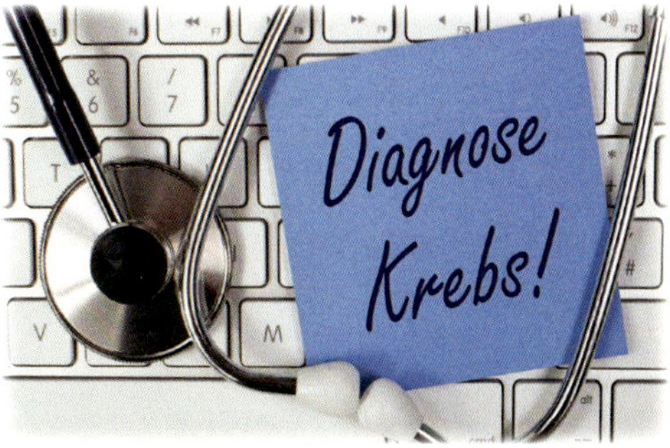

ACTIVITY 4

Give an answer!

1. Who drew up the flyer?
2. Who is the flyer aimed for?
3. What is not enough to diagnose breast cancer?
4. A patient's grandmother died of breast cancer and her mother found a lump in one of her breasts ten years ago. What would you advise such a patient?
5. If a woman finds a lump in one of her breasts. Does that mean that she has got breast cancer?
6. What kinds of tumours are there?
7. What will gynaecologists do in uncertain cases?
8. What will the staff of the surgery in the text give patients if they have any questions concerning the diagnosis of breast cancer?

Mrs. Patricia Rice found the flyer in the waiting room of her German consultant gynaecologist. She read it. She thinks to have found a very small but hard lump in one of her breasts. She is very worried because she has already read a lot about the dangers of breast cancer. She is so nervous that she does not even want to take a seat in the waiting room. With the flyer in her hand she walks up to the reception desk and speaks to the receptionist ...

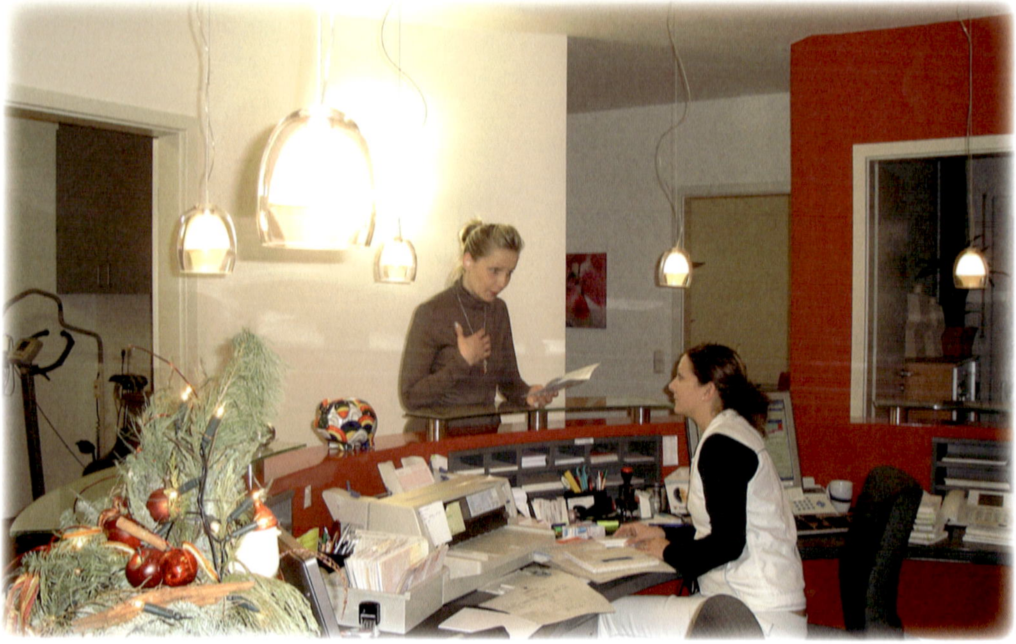

Mrs. Rice	Ah ... Excuse me. Have you got a minute?
Receptionist	Sure. How can I help you, madam?
Mrs. Rice	Well ... You know ... I examine my breasts regularly. A few days ago, I found a small but hard lump in my left breast. I visited our family doctor and he sent me here straight away. I'm so worried that I even can't sleep anymore.
Receptionist	I understand that you are worried. But those lumps are very often just harmless cysts. Don't assume the worst!
Mrs. Rice	But what will happen if it is **not** just a cyst?
Receptionist	To make absolutely sure what exactly it is, we will make a mammography, an ultrasound scan or even send you to a radiologist for a MRI of your breast.
Mrs. Rice	What do you mean by "mammography"?
Receptionist	It's an X-ray of your breasts.
Mrs. Rice	I'm so worried that I will lose a breast ...
Receptionist	Don't worry too much, Mrs. Rice. Nowadays, this only happens in rare cases. If it is a tumour, it doesn't mean that you will lose your breast!
Mrs. Rice	I really hope that it isn't anything serious.
Receptionist	I hope so too. Ah ... Is there a history of cancer in your family?
Mrs. Rice	No. None of our family ever had or died of cancer so far.
Receptionist	You see, that's a good reason to be optimistic!
Mrs. Rice	Well, I must say I'm quite relieved after talking to you! Thanks!
Receptionist	You're welcome Mrs. Rice. Oh, by the way, the doctor can see you now. Take a seat in consulting room 2. It's just at the end of the corridor ...

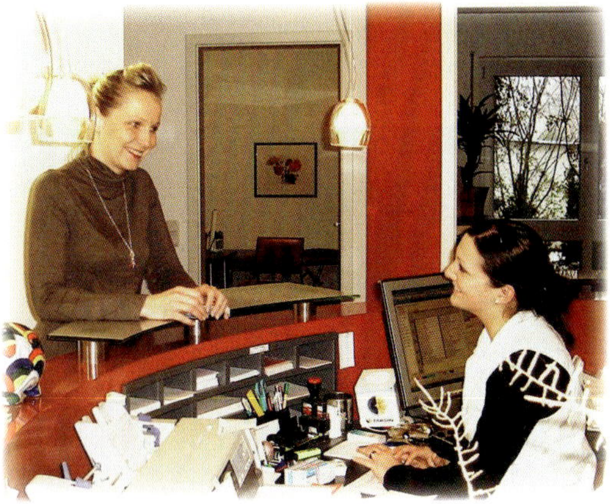

ACTIVITY 5

Find the words in the text and make a vocabulary list!

Handzettel	Facharzt für Gynäkologie	auf etwas zugehen
Anmeldung	sich wenden an (Person)	vor ein paar Tagen
gleich, sofort, umgehend	annehmen, vermuten	das Schlimmste
heutzutage	in sehr seltenen Fällen	das bedeutet nicht
verlieren	es ist nichts Ernstes	Ich hoffe es auch
Krebs-Vorgeschichte	keine/er/es	bisher
ein guter Grund	optimistisch sein	ziemlich erleichtert sein
Oh, übrigens ...	Sprechzimmer 2	Gang, Korridor

ACTIVITY 6

Answer the questions in English!

1. Where did Mrs. Rice find the flyer?
2. What did she find when she examined her breasts?
3. Why is she worried now?
4. She does not want to take a seat in the waiting room. Why?
5. What did her GP do, after she told him what she found in her breast?
6. Why is she not able to sleep anymore?
7. The assistant reassures her. How does she do that?
8. What will a gynaecologist do if he or she is uncertain?
9. What is a "mammography"?
10. The assistant tells Mrs. Rice not to worry too much about losing a breast. Why is there little reason to worry nowadays?
11. Is there a history of cancer in Mrs. Rice's family?
12. How does Mrs. Rice feel after talking to the doctor's assistant?
13. Where is consulting room 2?

UNIT 8

ACTIVITY 7

Ask your partner questions. Take turns!

1. Is there a history of cancer in your family?
2. Has anyone of your family ever died of cancer?
3. Do you regularly examine your breasts?
4. What about your mother? Does she do it?
5. Do you know what a "mammography" is?
6. Does it often happen nowadays that women lose one of their breasts because of breast cancer?
7. If a doctor diagnoses a tumour, does that mean that the person has got cancer?

ACTIVITY 8

Have this conversation with an English speaking patient!

Assistant	Patient
	1. Sie fragen die MFA, ob sie kurz Zeit für ein Gespräch hat.
2. Natürlich haben Sie kurz Zeit für die Patientin.	
	3. Sagen Sie ihr, dass Sie Ihre Brüste regelmäßig abtasten. Jetzt haben Sie einen kleinen aber harten Knoten entdeckt. Sie haben Angst, dass es ein Tumor sein könnte.
4. Beruhigen Sie die Patientin und weisen Sie sie darauf hin, dass es sich oft nur um harmlose Zysten handelt.	
	5. Sie möchten wissen, was wäre, falls es keine harmlose Zyste ist.
6. Sagen Sie ihr, dass man sie, um sicherzugehen, zum Radiologen schicken wird. Dort würde man eine Mammografie und/oder eine Ultraschalluntersuchung machen.	
	7. Fragen Sie, was eine „Mammografie“ ist.
8. Erklären Sie es kurz.	
	9. Sie haben Angst davor, eine Brust zu verlieren
10. Beruhigen Sie die Patientin und klären Sie darüber auf, wie groß dieses Risiko ist.	
	11. Reagieren Sie darauf.
12. Fragen Sie die Patientin, ob jemand in ihrer Familie bereits Krebs hatte.	
	13. Bejahen Sie dies. Sagen Sie, dass Ihre Großmutter an Brustkrebs starb.
14. Weisen Sie in diesem Falle auf ein erhöhtes Risiko hin. Machen Sie der Patientin aber dennoch Mut.	
	15. Bedanken Sie sich für das Gespräch. Drücken Sie Erleichterung aus.
16. Sie erwidern den Dank der Patientin und bitten Sie, sich in das Sprechzimmer 2 zu begeben.	
	17. Sie fragen, wo es ist.
18. Erklären Sie der Patientin, wo es sich befindet.	

EXTENDED VOCABULARY LIST	
aware (of)	bewusst, sich dessen bewusst sein
benign	gutartig
breast	Busen, Brust, Brüste
cancer	Karzinom, Krebs, bösartige Geschwulst
certain(ly)	sicher, sicherlich
clinical	klinisch, unpersönlich, steril
concern	Sorge, Angelegenheit, Konzern
concerning	betreffend, bezüglich, in Bezug auf
contain	enthalten, beinhalten
container	Behälter
cyst	Zyste
cystitis	Blasenentzündung
deal with	umgehen mit, zurecht kommen mit
diagnose	Diagnose, diagnostizieren
draw up	entwerfen
examine	prüfen, untersuchen, abtasten
experience	Erlebnis, Erfahrung
experienced	erfahren, sachkundig
female/male	weiblich/männlich
flyer	Handzettel, Flieger(in), Flyer
gynaecological	gynäkologisch
hesitate	zögern
hesitation	das Zögern, Unschlüssigkeit, Unentschlossenheit
leaflet	Prospekt, Faltblatt, Broschüre
loose	locker, lose, frei, ungebunden
lose	verlieren, einbüßen
lump	Knoten, Beule (Med.), Schwellung
MRI (Magnetic Resonance Imaging)	MRT, Magnetresonanz-Tomografie, Kernspintomografie
make sure	sichergehen, sich versichern
male/female	männlich/weiblich

UNIT 8

EXTENDED VOCABULARY LIST	
malignant	bösartig, maligne
mammography, mammogram	Mammografie
meaning	Bedeutung, Sinn;
none	keine/r/es
once/twice/three times	einmal/zweimal/dreimal
rare	selten, rar, ungewöhnlich
reassure	beruhigen, ein Gefühl der Sicherheit geben
regular(ly)	regelmäßig
so far	bisher, bislang, bis jetzt
staff	Personal, Mitarbeiter, Stab, Stock
straight away	sofort, gleich, umgehend
tumour	Geschwulst, Tumor
turn to	sich wenden an
uncertain	unklar, unsicher, ungewiss
vocation	Beruf
vocational college/school	Berufsschule, berufliche Schule
What's the meaning of ...?	Was heißt ...?
X-ray	Röntgenstrahl, Röntgenbild

9 THE STUDENT OF MUSIC

Miss Anna Sukova from Russia studies song at a German academy of music. Students from non-European Union countries are usually required to take out health insurance with a German health insurance company for the time of their studies in Germany. After about three month in Germany, Ms. Sukova is feeling very weak with circulatory trouble accompanied with bad coughing and sneezing. She decides to visit the general practitioner Dr. Astrid Kessler, whose surgery is located close to her academy. Ms. Sukova has not got an appointment. She speaks English quite well but her German is still poor. Kathrina, Dr. Kessler's assistant, is sitting at the reception desk ...

Ms. Sukova Guten Morgen.

Kathrina Guten Morgen. Was kann ich für Sie tun?

Ms. Sukova Mein Deutsch ist noch nicht so gut. Ah ... Can I speak English?

Kathrina No problem. What can I do for you?

Ms. Sukova I urgently need to see the doctor.

Kathrina Unfortunately, we are a bit busy today. Without an appointment you will have to wait for some time, I'm afraid. What's your problem?

Ms. Sukova I'm feeling terribly weak and seem to have no energy at all. I have had flu-like symptoms for a while too. I don't feel right at all. I even got diarrhoea and have to vomit now and then...

Kathrina Oh ... is it that bad? OK, let me see what I can do ... Have you got German health insurance or are you paying cash?

Ms. Sukova I have this medical card here...

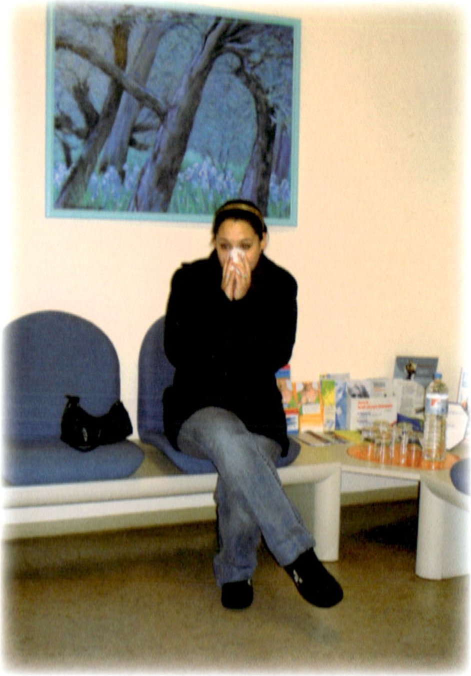

Kathrina That's great. May I have it please?

Ms. Sukova Sure, here you are

Kathrina (She looks at it and puts it into the card reader) ...
OK, Ms. Sukova, could you please take a seat in the waiting room. But, as I've just said, it may take a while.

Ms. Sukova No problem. Where's the waiting room?

Katharina Right opposite.

After Dr. Kessler has examined Ms. Sukova

Kathrina Just a moment, Ms. Sukova. I'll print out doctor Kessler's prescription and sick certificate for you. Here you are.

Ms. Sukova Where is the nearest pharmacy?

Kathrina Oh, there is a pharmacy just down the road at the crossroads. Go outside the building and then turn left. It's about 200 meters from here ...

Ms. Sukova Thanks a lot. Bye.

Kathrina You're welcome. Bye.

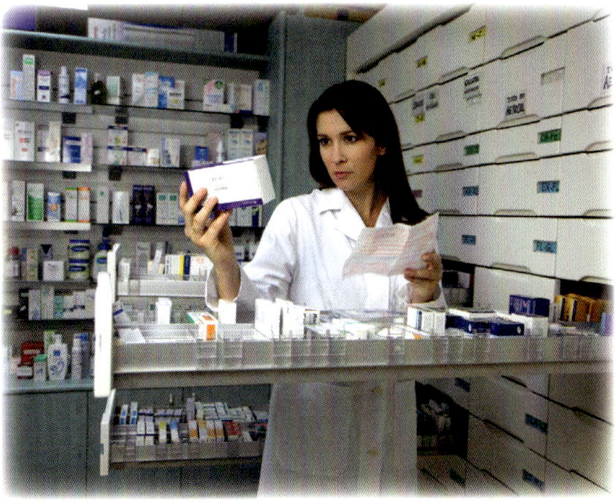

Will it hurt?

A woman is in a private beauty clinic to undergo breast aumentation.
She asks: "Will the surgery hurt me, doctor?"
The doctor replies: "Only when you receive my bill"

(to undergo = sich unterziehen; breast augmentation = Brustvergrößerung; to hurt = weh tun; reply = erwidern; only when = erst wenn; receive = erhalten; bill = Rechnung)

ACTIVITY 1

Find these words and expressions in the text and add them to your vocabulary list!

Musikstudent/in	Gesang studieren	Musikhochschule, Musik Akademie
Länder, die nicht der EU angehören	es wird von ihnen verlangt	eine Versicherung abschließen
Krankenversicherung (Unternehmen)	Kreislaufbeschwerden	verbunden mit
Husten und Niesen	er/sie/es liegt	nahe bei, in der Nähe von
schlecht, unzureichend	leider, unglücklicherweise	ein bisschen voll
sich schwach fühlen	überhaupt keine Energie haben	grippeähnliche Symptome
seit einiger Zeit	Durchfall, Diarrhö	brechen, erbrechen
hin und wieder	Krankenversicherung	KV-Karte
Kartenlesegerät	es wird eine Weile dauern	Wartezimmer
genau gegenüber	ausdrucken	Rezept, Verschreibung
Hier bitte!	nächstgelegene Apotheke	die Straße hinunter
an der Kreuzung	Gehen Sie nach draußen...	biegen Sie nach links ab
Vielen Dank!	Gern geschehen!	Tschüss

UNIT 9

ACTIVITY 2

Please, give an answer in English!

1. What kind of insurance do students from non-EU countries usually have take out?
2. Which health problems has Ms. Sukova got?
3. She visits Dr. Kessler's surgery. What might have been the reason why she chose Dr. Kessler's surgery?
4. Can Ms. Sukova speak German very well?
5. She has not got an appointment. Is that a problem?
6. Has Ms. Sukova got a medical card?
7. The doctor's assistant gave her a prescription. Where will she get the prescribed medicines from?
8. Describe Ms. Sukova's way to the pharmacy!

ACTIVITY 3

Tell a patient the way!

Go	round the corner down the hall/along the corridor downstairs upstairs through the door to the ground floor to the first floor to the fourth floor to the top floor
It's	opposite the reception across the road at the end of the corridor/hall
Take	the lift (UK) the elevator (US) the stairs (UK)/the stairway (US)
Turn	left/right
It's	the first door on the left the last door on the right in the basement/on the first floor

Make sentences in English!

Example: "Go upstairs, turn round the corner, then down/along the corridor. It's the third door on the left"

1. Gehen Sie die Treppe hinunter zum ersten Stock, dann nach links und dann den Gang entlang. Es ist die dritte Tür links.
2. Gehen Sie in die oberste Etage, dann durch die Tür und dann um die Ecke. Es ist die zweite Tür rechts.
3. Nehmen Sie den Lift nach oben zur dritten Etage, dann nach links. Gehen Sie den Gang entlang. Es ist die letzte Tür auf der linken Seite.
4. Sie finden den Raum im Kellergeschoss. Nehmen Sie den Lift, dann durch die Tür, den Gang entlang. Es ist die erste Tür rechts.
5. Um die Ecke, die Treppe hinunter, den Gang entlang, dann nach rechts.
6. Die Toilette ist am Ende des Ganges.
7. Das Labor ist gegenüber dem Behandlungsraum.
8. Das Wartezimmer ist auf der anderen Seite des Ganges.

ACTIVITY 4

Say it in English!

1. Ich habe Durchfall und muss hin und wieder erbrechen.
2. Frau Sukova hat keinen Termin.
3. Ihr Deutsch ist noch sehr schlecht.
4. Sie braucht dringend einen Arzt.
5. Lassen Sie mich sehen, was ich tun kann!
6. Darf ich Ihre Krankenversicherungskarte haben?
7. Hier, bitte!
8. Einen Moment bitte!
9. Wo bekomme ich die verschriebenen Medikamente?
10. In der Apotheke.
11. Wo ist sie?
12. Gehen Sie nach draußen und biegen Sie nach rechts ab.
13. Gehen Sie die Straße hinunter.
14. Die Apotheke befindet sich an der Kreuzung.
15. Es sind nur etwa 100 Meter von hier.
16. Vielen Dank! – Gern geschehen/Bitte!

A man goes to the doctor and says to him: „It hurts when I press here" (He presses one side of his body)
"And it hurts when I press there" (He presses the other side)
"And here" (He presses his leg)
"And here, and here and here..." (He presses everywhere)
The doctor examined him all over and finally found the reason why:
You've got a broken finger!"

ACTIVITY 5

You are a family doctor's assistant. Give advice!

Assistant	Patient
	1. Sie sprechen sehr schlecht Deutsch. Sie fragen, ob Sie auch Englisch sprechen können.
2. Sie bejahen und fragen, was Sie für den Patienten/die Patientin tun können.	
	3. Sie brauchen dringend einen Arzt. Schildern Sie Ihre Symptome.
4. Sagen Sie, dass man ohne Termin normalerweise einige Zeit warten muss. Aber der Patient/die Patientin hat Glück. Heute ist nicht viel los.	

Assistant	Patient
	5. Sie reagieren erleichtert.
6. Fragen Sie ihn/sie, ob er/sie eine KV-Karte einer deutschen Versicherung besitzt oder bar bezahlt.	
	7. Sie sind Student/Studentin und haben eine deutsche KV-Karte.
8. Verlangen Sie höflich die Zahlung der Praxisgebühr.	
	9. Sie kommen der Aufforderung nach und bezahlen.
10. Fragen Sie höflich, ob Sie die KV-Karte sehen könnten.	
	11. Sie kommen der Aufforderung nach

Back to our story ...

After Ms. Sukova's treatment is finished, she leaves Dr. Kessler's surgery and walks down the road to the pharmacy at the crossroads. There she gets all the prescribed medicines. About 30 minutes later she enters the surgery once again ...

Ms. Sukova Hello again.

Assistant Oh, Ms. Sukova, did you forget something or do you need another appointment?

Ms. Sukova No, I don't. I just wondered if you could help me with a language problem.

Assistant Sure. What's your problem?

Ms. Sukova Well, I have just been to the pharmacy ... (She keeps coughing and sneezing)

Assistant You sound like you might be getting a really bad flu. There is a flu bug going around at the moment, you know ...

Ms. Sukova I know. A lot of my friends already got it. Well, here I got the medicines which Dr. Kessler prescribed for my flu.
The problem is, I can't read the dosage instructions. No one could speak English at the pharmacy and translate the instructions for me.

Assistant Can I have a look? (She looks at the dosage instructions for the cough medicine ...). Well, it says her: "Take three to four capsules a day after meals. Do not take them on an empty stomach or with other medication. Swallow the capsules with water. The capsules should not be taken for any longer than 4 days.
If the symptoms still persist, please see your doctor again. This medicine may cause drowsiness. Side effects: The medicine can cause stomach and intestinal troubles. In rare cases sickness".

Ms. Sukova	Ah ... well. Thank you.
Assistant	Anything else?
Ms. Sukova	Oh, yes. I got this mixture here for my bronchitis ... (She shows her a small bottle.)
Assistant	Let me see ... Well, these drops should be taken regularly. Take half a tablespoonful, which is 10 to 15 drops, every 4 hours. Take them until all symptoms have disappeared. The drops should be taken before meals.
Ms. Sukova	Fine. There's one more problem. Another doctor prescribed me an antibiotic last week. I have taken the tablets for 5 days and all symptoms have gone. Can I stop taking them?
Assistant	No, never do that! It is very important to take them all. If you stop taking them too soon, it may happen that some of the bacteria survive and start spreading again. You may run the risk that the antibiotic will not work the next time you have to take some.
Ms. Sukova	Thank you so much for your assistance.
Assistant	Oh, no problem! It was a pleasure helping you.

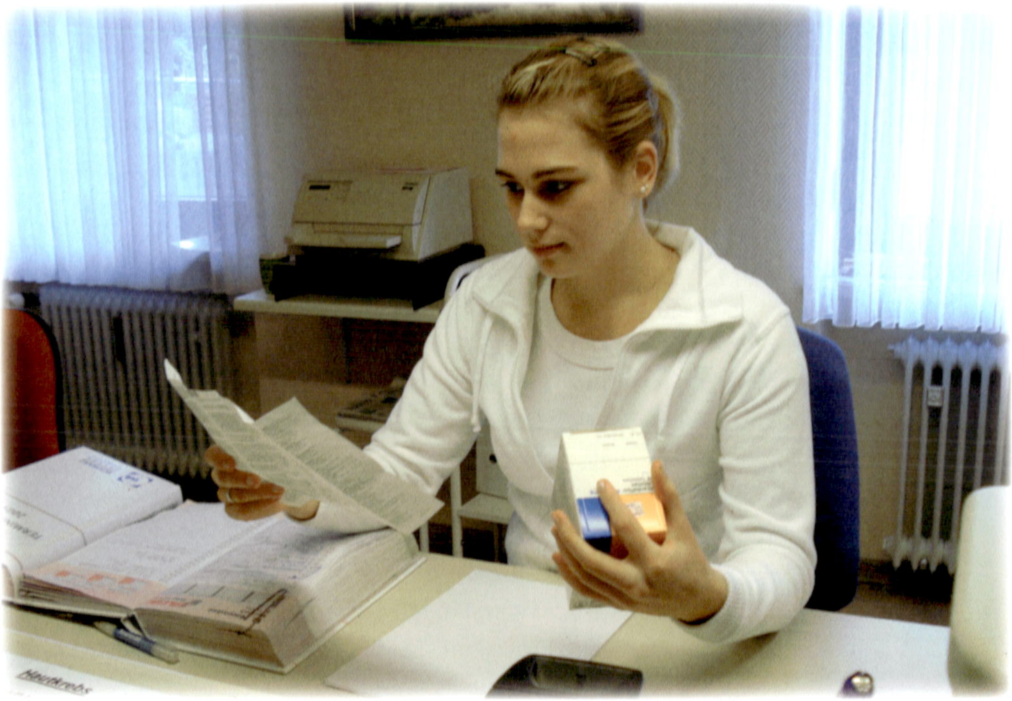

ACTIVITY 6

Find these words in the text and add them to your vocabulary list!

wann auch immer, sobald	sich etwas fragen	Apotheke
es hört sich an wie ...	Grippebazillus	die Dosierung, Dosis
Beipackzettel, Dosierungsschema	Hustenmittel	Hier steht ...
Kapseln	auf leeren Magen	schlucken, nehmen
nicht länger als	noch andauern	Müdigkeit, Schläfrigkeit
Nebenwirkung	Magen-Darm-Beschwerden	in seltenen Fällen
Übelkeit	Noch etwas?	Mischung, Mixtur
Tropfen	regelmäßig nehmen	ein halber Esslöffel voll
verschwinden	Mahlzeit	Antibiotikum
Nehmen Sie alle	mindestens	Bakterien
überleben	(sich) ausbreiten	das Risiko eingehen
wirken, arbeiten	nächstes Mal	Vergnügen

ACTIVITY 7

How would you translate the following dosage instructions for an English speaking patient?

1. Schlucken Sie die Tabletten mit Wasser.
2. Nehmen Sie täglich 3–4 Kapseln.
3. Nehmen Sie die Tabletten nicht länger als 5 Tage lang ein.
4. Die Tropfen sollten regelmäßig alle 2 Stunden eingenommen werden.
5. Das Antibiotikum sollte nicht auf nüchternen Magen eingenommen werden.
6. Das Medikament kann Müdigkeit verursachen.
7. Sollten die Symptome andauern, suchen Sie bitte einen Arzt auf.
8. Nehmen Sie drei Mal täglich einen halben Teelöffel voll.
9. Beenden Sie die Einnahme von Antibiotika nicht zu früh.
10. Nehmen Sie das Medikament nicht (zusammen) mit anderen Medikamenten ein.
11. Die Tabletten sollten vor den Mahlzeiten eingenommen werden
12. Nehmen Sie das Medikament mindestens 7 Tage lang ein.
13. Nehmen Sie die Kapseln (solange) bis alle Symptome verschwunden sind.
14. In seltenen Fällen kann das Medikament Übelkeit verursachen.
15. Nehmen Sie alle 2 Stunden 20 bis 30 Tropfen ein.

ACTIVITY 8

Ask your partner questions!

1. Which symptoms are typical if you have got flu?
2. How do you deal with patients who come without an appointment?
3. A patient has got flu. What would you advise him/her to do for it?
4. A family doctor thinks that his/her patient has got a very special medical problem. Where will the family doctor probably send the patient?
5. Should you stop taking an antibiotic as soon as all symptoms have gone/disappeared?
6. Why should you never stop taking antibiotics too early?

EXTENDED VOCABULARY LIST	
advantage	Vorteil
antibiotic	Antibiotikum, antibiotisch
Anything else?	(Gibt es) noch etwas?
basement	Kellergeschoss, Untergeschoss
bug	Bazillus, Käfer, Fehler (Software)
by now	mittlerweile, bis jetzt
capsules	Kapseln
cough medicine	Hustenmittel
coughing	husten
disappear	verschwinden, entschwinden
dosage	Dosierung, Dosis
drowsiness	Müdigkeit, Schläfrigkeit
drowsy	müde, schläfrig
food	Essen, Nahrungsmittel, Futter
hall (US), corridor (UK)	Flur
instruction	Anweisung, Vorschrift
intestinal troubles	Darmbeschwerden
kind of	(eine) Art (von)

EXTENDED VOCABULARY LIST	
meanwhile	inzwischen, zwischenzeitlich, unterdessen
medication	Arznei, Medikament(e), Medikation
medicine	Medizin, Arznei
medicine for (not against!!!)	Arznei für bzw. gegen
minor	klein, geringfügig, unbedeutend
offer	anbieten, bieten, Angebot
once again	noch einmal, wieder einmal
persist	andauern, fortbestehen
pharmacist (US), chemist (UK)	Apotheker
pills	Pillen, Tabletten
pleasure	Vergnügen, Freude
prescription **recipe**	Verschreibung Kochrezept
probably	wahrscheinlich, vermutlich
prove	beweisen, nachweisen
quarter (of a year)	Quartal, Vierteljahr
reader	Leser, Lesegerät
regular(ly)	regelmäßig
run	rennen, laufen, eingehen (Risiko)
safe	sicher, Safe
save	sparen, retten
sickness	Übelkeit, Erkrankung, Krankheit
side effect	Nebenwirkung, Nebenerscheinung
sound like	sich anhören wie
spoonful	ein Löffel voll
spread	ausbreiten, ausstrecken
stomach troubles	Magenbeschwerden
table spoon/tea spoon	Esslöffel/Teelöffel
take out	abschließen (Versicherung) herausnehmen
take part in	teilnehmen an, mitmachen bei
top floor	oberstes Stockwerk/Etage/Geschoss

EXTENDED VOCABULARY LIST	
turn	Reihenfolge, Kurve, abbiegen, drehen
unfortunately	leider, bedauerlicherweise
upstairs/downstairs	oben/unten
vomit, to throw up	erbrechen, brechen
wonder	erstaunt sein, sich fragen, sich wundern, Wunder
work	wirken, funktionieren, arbeiten

A woman is calling the receptionist of a hospital and says: "Hello, I want to know if a patient is getting better."

The receptionist replies: "What is the patient's name and room number?"

The woman says: "She's Sarah Finkel, in room 302."

The receptionist says: "Oh, Mrs. Finkel is doing very well. Her blood pressure is fine and if she continues this improvement, Doctor Frank is going to send her home on Tuesday."

The woman says: "Thank God! That's wonderful! Oh, that's fantastic!"

"You seem to be a very close friend or family member?" the receptionist asks.

"No", she answers, "**I am** Sarah Finkel. I called you because Doctor Frank never tells me a word!"

(reply = erwidern; to continue an improvement = weitere Fortschritte machen; close friend = enger Freund; family member = Familienmitglied)

10 AN ALLERGY

Miss Catherine McLaren, a young Canadian woman from Quebec, booked a two-week holiday trip around France and Germany. It is spring time. Catherine never suffered from an allergy so far. However, since she came to Germany she started wheezing, sneezing and coughing. Her nose is sometimes blocked and sometimes runny. Her eyes are watery and itchy. She assumes that she might be hypersensitive to something. Before they left Canada, Catherine took out travel insurance which also covers expenses for medical treatment abroad. The receptionist at their hotel advised her to visit the surgery of the consultant dermatologist and allergist, Dr. Andreas Lehmann. She enters his surgery and walks up to the reception desk ...

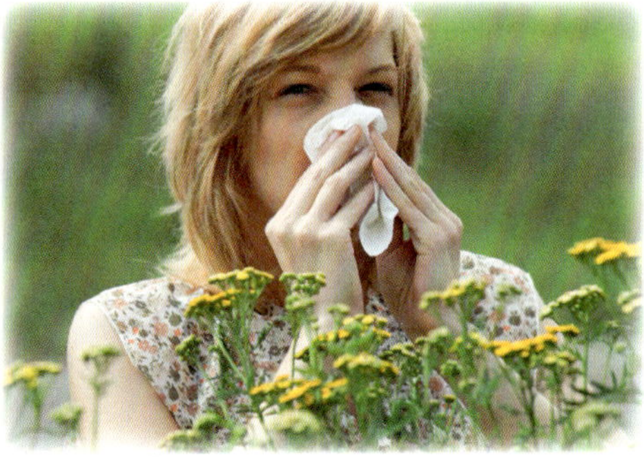

Receptionist Was kann ich für Sie tun?

Catherine Ah ... Do you speak English?

Receptionist Yes, a little.

Catherine Oh, good. I've got a bit of a problem. (She wheezes and sneezes)

Receptionist It looks like you've got some kind of an allergy ...

Catherine I think so, too. That's why I came here. Just to find out.

Receptionist Do you have an appointment?

Catherine No, I haven't.

Receptionist Well, you are lucky. We are not very busy today. You may have to wait but it won't take long. Could I have your name, please?

Catherine My name is McLaren. Catherine McLaren. I'm a tourist from Quebec, Canada.

Receptionist Could you please put your personal details here on this form and sign this fee agreement. I'm afraid, I will have to ask you to pay in cash.

Catherine Oh, that's no problem. I've got private health insurance.

After Dr. Lehmann has seen her

Assistant Would you please come along to the treatment room, Ms. McLaren? We will do an allergy test now.

Catherine What do you think it might be?

Assistant Oh, it could be anything. You might be allergic to animal hair, pollen, fruits, such as apples, cherries, kiwis or pears. You might also be allergic to nuts, such as hazelnuts, walnuts, almonds or peanuts and lots more.
But, looking at the symptoms you have, it looks like a pollen allergy or hay fever, as some people also call it. Birch pollen, for example, can cause real problems here in Germany.

Catherine I tried a nasal spray, but it didn't help. What can I do?

Assistant Well, taking antihistamines may help to control the symptoms. The best, however, would be a desensitization course to make you less sensitive to the things which cause your allergy.

Catherine I could try that when I'll be back in Canada ...

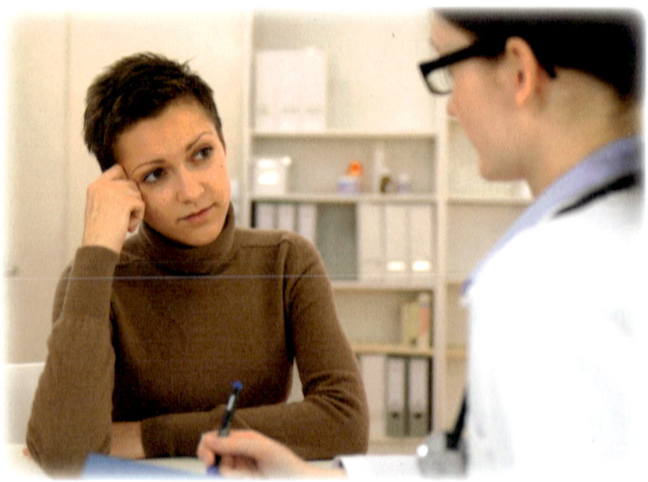

ACTIVITY 1

Please, find the English words in the text and add them to your vocabulary list!

Frühlingszeit	an etwas leiden	bisher
Jedoch ...	sie begann zu keuchen	niesen
husten	verstopft	meine Nase läuft
wässerig	juckend	es könnte sein
könnte sein	typisch sein für	Reiseversicherung abschließen

die Ausgaben decken	medizinische Behandlung	im Ausland
jemand riet mir...	Facharzt für Hautkrankheiten, Dermatologe, Hautarzt	Allergologe
auf die Anmeldung zugehen	ein kleines Problem haben	irgendeine Allergie
Das glaube ich auch!	deswegen, deshalb	Glück haben
sehr voll sein (Praxis)	es dauert lange	persönliche Angaben
unterschreiben	Honorarvereinbarung	Krankenversicherung
Kommen Sie mit!	allergisch (reagieren) auf	Tierhaar(e)
Blütenstaub, Pollen	Birnen	Haselnüsse
Walnüsse	Mandeln	Heuschnupfen
Birkenpollen	Nasenspray	Antihistamin Tabletten/ Pillen
die Symptome beeinflussen	Desensibilisierung	weniger sensibel machen

ACTIVITY 2

Answer these questions in English!

1. Why has Ms. McLaren come to Germany?
2. Has Ms. McLaren ever suffered from an allergy?
3. Which symptoms has she got since she came to Germany?
4. What does her boyfriend think?
5. Are Ms. McLaren's medical expenses covered here in Germany?
6. What kind of medical specialist is Dr. Andreas Lehmann?
7. Ms. McLaren is wheezing, sneezing and coughing. What does Dr. Lehmann's assistant guess what it might be?
8. Did Ms. McLaren book a medical appointment with Dr. Lehmann?
9. Why is Ms. McLaren lucky?
10. The doctor's assistant asks Ms. McLaren to sign something. What is it?
11. Why does the assistant ask Ms. McLaren to come along to the treatment room?
12. The assistant lists up things which people can be allergic to. Which things are they?
13. Ms. McLaren already tried out something to fight her wheezing and sneezing. What was it?
14. What about antihistamines? Would they help?
15. What can allergists do to make people less sensitive to the things that cause an allergy?

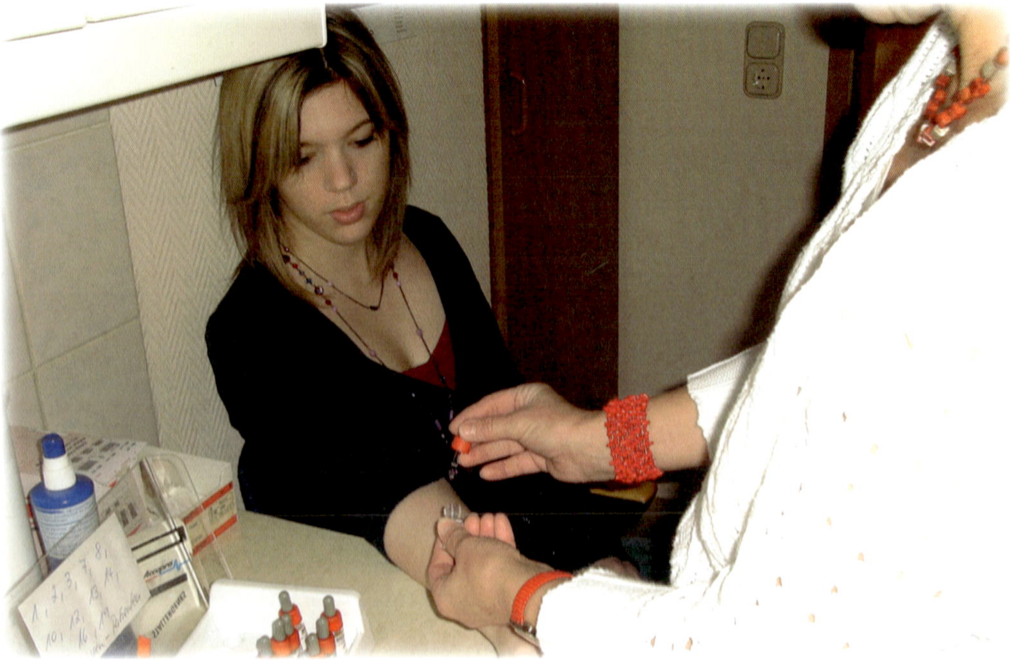

ACTIVITY 3

Can you say it in English!

1. Im Frühling und Sommer leide ich immer an Heuschnupfen.
2. Heuschnupfen ist eine Pollenallergie.
3. Manche Menschen hatten noch nie eine Allergie.
4. Menschen, die an Heuschnupfen leiden, husten, niesen, keuchen, haben eine laufende oder verstopfte Nase und wässrige, juckende Augen.
5. Ich glaube, es könnte eine Allergie sein.
6. Für meinen Auslandsaufenthalt habe ich eine Reiseversicherung abgeschlossen.
7. Sie deckt auch die Aufwendungen für medizinische Behandlung.
8. Dr. Lehmann ist Dermatologe und Allergologe.
9. Sie haben irgendeine Allergie.
10. Das glaube ich auch!
11. Ich kam (her), um es herauszufinden.
12. Sie haben Glück. Die Praxis ist heute nicht sehr voll.
13. Es wird nicht lange dauern.
14. Könnten Sie hier ein paar persönliche Angaben machen?
15. Unterschreiben Sie bitte diese Honorarvereinbarung/Kostenübernahmeerklärung.
16. Darf ich Sie bitten, bar zu zahlen?
17. Ich bin privat krankenversichert.
18. Kommen Sie bitte mit!
19. Was meinen Sie, was es sein könnte?
20. Es könnte alles Mögliche sein.
21. Ich bin allergisch auf Tierhaare.

22. Nein, ich bin nicht allergisch auf Nüsse.
23. Das sieht nach einer Pollenallergie aus.
24. Birkenpollen können echte Probleme verursachen.
25. Wenn man Heuschnupfen hat, hilft ein Nasenspray nicht viel.
26. Antihistamine jedoch können die Symptomatik beeinflussen.
27. Ich möchte eine Hypo- bzw. Desensibilisierung durchführen lassen.

ACTIVITY 4

Ask your partner questions. Take turns!

1. What is "hay fever"?
2. Can you list up things which some people are allergic to?
3. How can antihistamines help?
4. Would you try a desensitization course if you had a really bad allergy?
5. Which symptoms are typical if you suffer from hay fever?
6. Why are there warnings on many products saying: "This product contains nuts or traces of nuts"?

ACTIVITY 5

You are a dermatologist's assistant. Make this conversation with an English speaking tourist!

Assistant	Tourist
	1. Sagen Sie, dass Sie, seit Sie sich in Deutschland aufhalten, niesen und husten müssen.
2. Fragen Sie die Touristin nach weiteren Symptomen.	
	3. Ihre Nase ist dauernd verstopft und läuft.
4. Sie stellen fest, dass die Touristin feuchte Augen hat. Fragen Sie, ob ihre Augen jucken.	
	5. Bejahen Sie dies und betonen Sie, dass sich die Symptome verschlimmern.
6. Erwähnen Sie, dass Dr. Lehmann ein erfahrener Allergologe ist.	
	7. Fragen Sie, ob es irgendeine Allergie sein könnte.

Assistant	Tourist
8. Sie vermuten, dass es sich tatsächlich um eine Allergie handeln könnte.	
	9. Fragen Sie, auf welche Dinge Menschen allergisch reagieren können.
10. Zählen Sie einige Dinge auf.	
	11. Fragen Sie, was man dagegen tun könnte.
12. Weisen Sie darauf hin, dass im Falle eines Heuschnupfens ein Nasenspray nicht wirklich hilft. Antihistamine können die Symptome jedoch entscheidend beeinflussen.	
	13. Fragen Sie, was man tun kann, um weniger sensibel auf Allergieauslöser zu reagieren.
14. Sagen Sie, dass es am besten wäre, eine Desensibilisierung durchführen zu lassen. Es müssen jedoch erst die Ergebnisse des Allergietests abgewartet werden.	

EXTENDED VOCABULARY LIST

abroad	im Ausland
actually	eigentlich, übrigens, tatsächlich
birch	Birke
come along	mitkommen, folgen
cough	Husten, husten
cover	bedecken, decken, einwickeln, decken, Decke, Überzug
fight	bekämpfen, Kampf
fruit	Obst
fruits	Früchte
itch	Juckreiz, das Jucken; Lust auf (for)
itchy	juckend
kind of	eine Art von, irgendwie, sozusagen
list up	aufzählen, auflisten
might	könnte vielleicht, dürfte, Macht, Gewalt, Stärke, Kraft
nasal	nasal, näselnd

EXTENDED VOCABULARY LIST	
pollen	Pollen, Blütenstaub
sensible	vernünftig (Nicht verwechseln mit „sensibel"!!)
sensitive	empfindlich, sensibel, einfühlsam
since	seit, seitdem, seither, zuvor, da, weil
sneeze	niesen
traces	Spuren
try out	ausprobieren
walk up to	auf etwas zugehen/zulaufen, hinaufgehen
warning	Warnhinweis, Warnung, Mahnung
wheeze	keuchen, pfeifender Ton

A seven-year-old girl told her mom "A boy in my class asked me to play doctor."

"Oh dear", the mother nervously sighed. "What did he do to you, honey?"

"Nothing. He made me wait for two hours and then sent me a bill for 400 Euros."

(mom = Mama; Oh dear! = Du liebe Güte!; nervous = nervös; to sigh = seufzen; to make someone wait = jemanden warten lassen; bill = Rechnung)

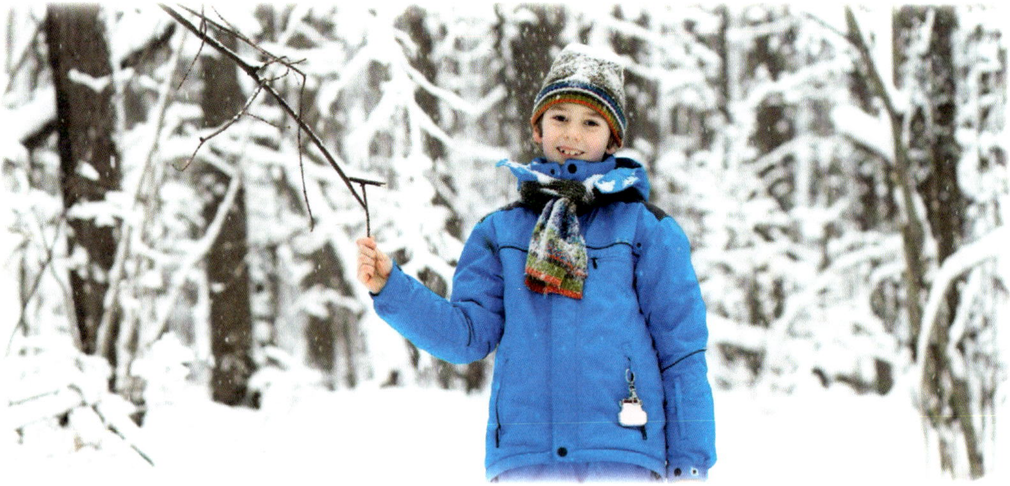

11 A COMPLETE PHYSICAL CHECK-UP

Miss Anna Sukova, the young Russian student has now finished her studies at the academy of music. She got her first engagement as a soprano singer at a German opera house for the current opera season. However, she has been feeling ill for some time now. She called the surgery of the general practitioner, Dr. Astrid Kessler, to get an appointment for a complete physical check-up. It is Monday morning, 8.23 a.m. Ms. Sukova is entering the surgery and walking up to the reception desk ...

Ms. Sukova Guten Morgen.

Receptionist Guten Morgen. Was kann ich für Sie tun?

Ms. Sukova I already know that you speak English. My German is still far from perfect, you know. I hope you don't mind me speaking English. My name is Sukova. Anna Sukova. I have an appointment for a check-up.

Receptionist Let me have a look. Ah yes ... for 8.30, right? Could you please fill in this form? We need a few personal details from you.

Ms. Sukova Sure. But, I suppose you already got all the details in your computer.

Receptionist Ah, I can remember you now. You were here about two years ago, weren't you?

Ms. Sukova That's right.

Receptionist May I have your medical card?

Ms. Sukova I have private health insurance now. I'll pay cash.

Receptionist Good. Could you please take a seat in the waiting room? It will take a few minutes. Oh, I forgot to ask: Have you got an empty stomach?

Ms. Sukova Yes, I have.

4 minutes later

Assistant Ms. Sukova? Could you please take a seat in consulting room 1 for the physical examination? It's just over there. Dr. Kessler will be with you in a minute. After Dr. Kessler has examined you, please go to room 2 for an ultrasound scan of your internal organs.

Ms. Sukova Will the doctor examine my pancreas too? You know, last year it caused me a lot of trouble.

Assistant Yes, we do an examination of your pancreas too, as well as an examination of your liver, kidneys, stomach, intestines and your gallbladder. We also make an electrocardiogram.

Ms. Sukova Fine.

Assistant When the doctor is finished with her examinations, please take a seat in the lab. That's the room over there.

The examination by the doctor is finished. Ms. Sukova is in the lab now

Assistant I will take the blood specimen now. Can I have one of your arms? Could you please take off your jumper and roll up the sleeve of your blouse? – That's perfect. One more thing I need from you: Could you please go to the lavatory afterwards? We also need a urine specimen. You will find a plastic cup with your name on it in the lavatory. Please, leave the cup in the lavatory and place it on the sill of the wooden window there.

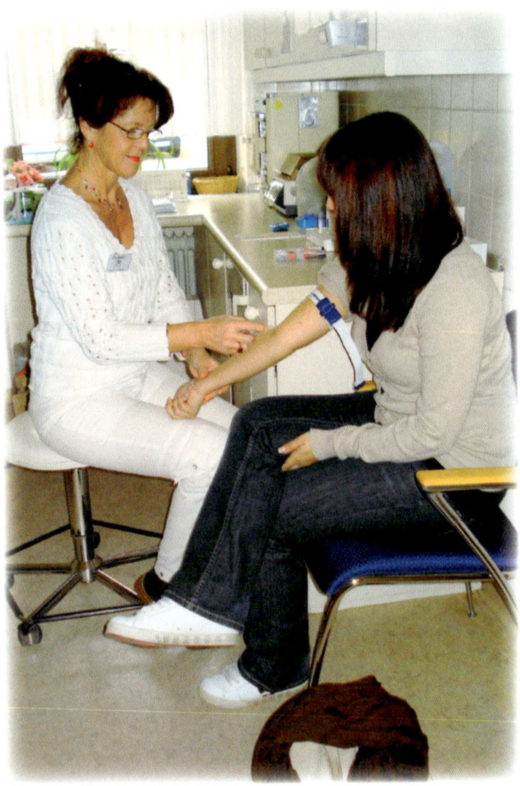

Ms. Sukova Alright.

Assistant In about three days, the results of the blood test will be back from the lab to which we'll send the blood specimen. Make another appointment in about three days. Then the doctor will talk to you about the lab results.

ACTIVITY 1

Find the words and expressions in the text and add them to your vocabulary list!

vollständig, komplett	körperliche Untersuchung	Verpflichtung, Engagement
Sopranistin	Opernhaus	laufende Opernsaison
seit einiger Zeit	nichts dagegen haben	private KV
nüchtern sein	Pankreas	sie verursachte mir
viele Probleme	Gallenblase	Blut abnehmen
hochkrempeln	die Ärmel	Noch etwas ...
danach, hinterher	Urinprobe	Plastikbecher
etwas platzieren, hinstellen	Fensterbank	Holzfenster
in zirka/ungefähr drei Tagen	einen weiteren Termin	die Laborergebnisse

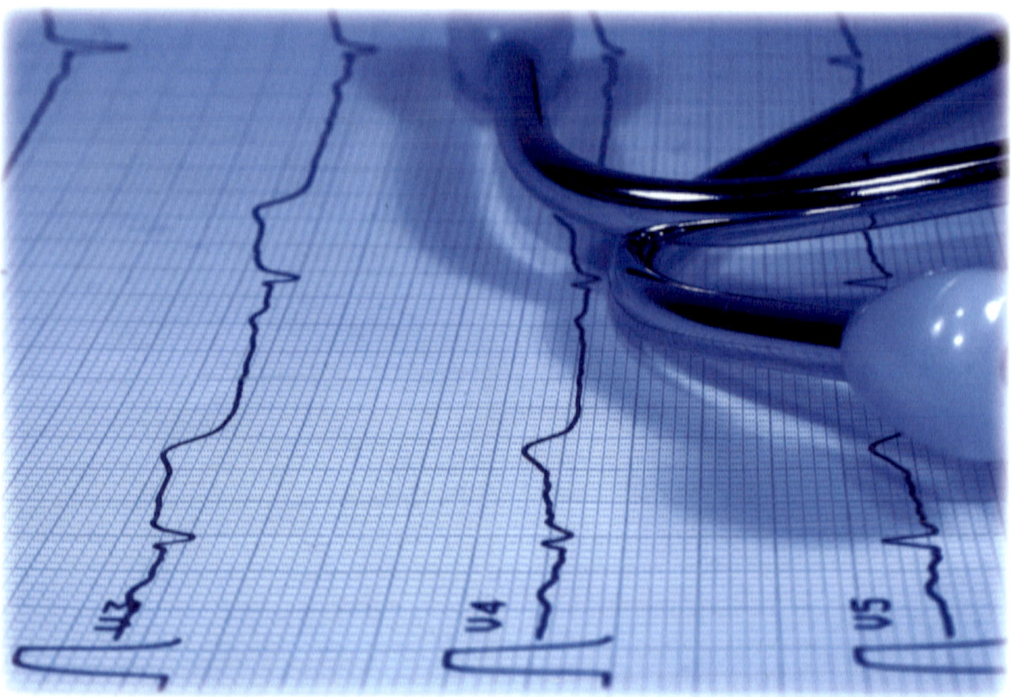

ACTIVITY 2

Please answer these questions in English!

1. What is Ms. Sukova doing in Germany?
2. Why did she call the surgery?
3. For what time and day has Ms. Sukova got an appointment?
4. What does the doctor's assistant need from Ms. Sukova?
5. What is very important, if you have a blood specimen taken?
6. Which rooms in the surgery will Ms. Sukova have to go to?
7. Why is Ms. Sukova interested in having her pancreas examined?
8. Which internal organs does Dr. Kessler usually examine?
9. How can a doctor find out if a patient's heart works properly?
10. Why does the assistant ask Ms. Sukova to go to the lab?
11. The assistant also needs a urine specimen too. She gives Ms. Sukova a few instructions. Which?
12. What will happen in about three day's time?
13. Why should Ms. Sukova make another appointment in about three days?

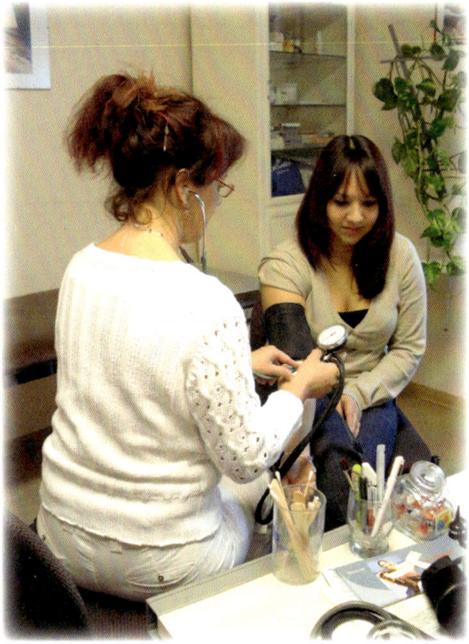

ACTIVITY 3

Can you say it in English?

1. Ich fühle mich (die ganze Zeit schon) unwohl/krank.
2. Sie sollten sich einen Termin für eine umfassende körperliche Untersuchung geben lassen.
3. Mir wurde gesagt, dass Sie Englisch sprechen.
4. Frau Sukova studierte Gesang.
5. Lassen Sie mich einmal nachsehen!
6. Ich habe Ihre Daten bereits in meinem Computer.
7. Ich kann mich an Sie erinnern!
8. Ich bin privat krankenversichert.
9. Ich benötige ein paar persönliche Angaben von Ihnen.
10. Nehmen Sie bitte im Wartezimmer Platz.
11. Sind Sie nüchtern?

12. Es wird ein paar Minuten dauern.
13. Nehmen Sie bitte im Zimmer 2 Platz.
14. Wo ist es?
15. Gleich da drüben.
16. Dr. Kessler wird eine Ultraschalluntersuchung Ihrer inneren Organe durchführen.
17. Die Nieren, die Leber, der Darm, die Gallenblase, der Blinddarm, der Magen und die Bauchspeicheldrüse sind in Ordnung.
18. Kommen Sie bitte mit. Wir machen jetzt (noch) ein EKG.
19. Könnten Sie danach im Labor Platz nehmen?
20. Wo ist das Labor?
21. Es ist das Zimmer dort drüben.
22. Dort werde ich (Ihnen) Blut abnehmen.
23. Könnten Sie bitte Ihren Ärmel hochkrempeln?
24. Ich benötige noch etwas von Ihnen.
25. Wir brauchen eine Urinprobe von Ihnen.
26. Könnten Sie bitte zur Toilette gehen?
27. Dort finden Sie einen Plastikbecher mit Ihrem Namen darauf.
28. Stellen Sie ihn auf das Fensterbrett.
29. In etwa drei Tagen werden wir die Ergebnisse haben/die Laborergebnisse haben.
30. Wir schicken das Blut in ein Labor.
31. Am Donnerstag wird der Arzt die Ergebnisse mit Ihnen besprechen.

ACTIVITY 4

Have a conversation with an English speaking patient!

Assistant	Patient
1. Eine Patientin steht vor der Anmeldung. Sie grüßen und fragen auf Deutsch, wie Sie ihr helfen können.	
	2. Ihnen wurde gesagt, dass in dieser Praxis auch Englisch gesprochen wird. Sie sprechen kein Deutsch. Sie stellen sich vor und sagen, dass Sie um 9:45 Uhr einen Termin für einen Check-up haben.
3. Sie sehen in das Terminbuch und bestätigen dies. Da Sie einige Angaben von der Patientin benötigen, bitten Sie sie, ein Formular auszufüllen.	
	4. Sie füllen das Formular aus.
5. Sie erkundigen sich, ob und wie die Patientin versichert ist.	
	6. Sie sagen, dass Sie privat krankenversichert sind und bar zahlen.
7. Sie fragen, ob die Patientin nüchtern ist.	

Assistant	Patient
	8. Sie bejahen.
9. Sie bitten die Patientin, im Wartezimmer Platz zu nehmen. Es wird noch ein wenig dauern.	
	10. Sie fragen, wo sich das Wartezimmer befindet.
11. Sie erklären, wo es sich befindet und sagen ihr, dass Sie sie aufrufen werden, wenn es soweit ist.	

About 15 minutes later

Assistant	Patient
Sie rufen die Patientin auf und bitten sie, im Sprechzimmer 1 Platz zu nehmen.	

After the examination by the doctor

Assistant	Patient
1. Sie bitten die Patientin, sich in Raum 3 zu einer Ultraschalluntersuchung zu begeben.	
	2. Sie würden gerne wissen, welche Organe üblicherweise untersucht werden.
3. Sie geben Auskunft und sagen ihr, dass sie nach der Untersuchung im Labor Platz nehmen soll.	

In the lab

Assistant	Patient
1. Sagen Sie der Patientin, dass Sie ihr jetzt Blut abnehmen werden und sie daher einen Arm freimachen soll. Danach wird noch ein EKG gemacht.	
	2. Erwidern Sie etwas.
3. Sie benötigen von der Patientin auch eine Urinprobe. Sie soll zur Toilette gehen. Dort findet sie ein Gefäß dafür. Sagen Sie ihr, wo sie das Gefäß hinstellen soll.	
	4. Erkundigen Sie sich, wann Sie mit den Ergebnissen rechnen können.
5. Dies wird in etwa 3 Tagen der Fall sein. Bitten Sie die Patientin, sich einen Termin in etwa 3 bis 4 Tagen geben zu lassen. Der Arzt wird die Ergebnisse dann mit ihr besprechen.	

EXTENDED VOCABULARY LIST	
another	ein/e weitere/r/es, noch ein/e
appendix	Blinddarm
as well as	wie auch, so gut wie, sowohl als auch
blouse	Bluse
check-up	gründliche Untersuchung, genaue Nachprüfung, Vorsorgeuntersuchung
physical check-up	körperliche Untersuchung, Hinweis: In der Umgangssprache wird so eine Untersuchung häufig kurz als „a physical" bezeichnet.
consultation	Rücksprache, Besprechung, (ärztliche) Beratung
consulting hours	Sprechzeit, Sprechstunden
consulting room	Sprechzimmer
cup	Becher, Tasse, Pokal
current	laufend, aktuell
finished (be)	fertig sein, erledigt sein
(be) far from	weit von etwas entfernt sein
jacket	Jacke, Jackett
jumper, sweater	Pullover
lab (Kurzform von *laboratory*)	Labor,
lavatory **restroom** **toilet**	Toilette (UK) Toilette (US) UK and US
(to) mind	etwas dagegen haben
pancreas	Pankreas, Bauchspeicheldrüse
place	platzieren, hinstellen, Ort
roll up	hochkrempeln, hinaufrollen
season	Saison, Jahreszeit
sill	(Fenster-)Sims, Fensterbank, Türschwelle
skirt	Rock
sleeve	Ärmel
suppose	annehmen, vermuten
take off	ablegen, ausziehen (Kleidung), starten, wegnehmen

An elderly man visits his family doctor and after a thorough examination, the doctor tells him "I have good news and bad news. What would you like to hear first?"

Patient: Well, give me the bad news first.

Doctor: You have cancer. I estimate that you have about two years left.

Patient: Oh no! That's awful! In two years time my life will be over??? What good news could you tell me after this?

Doctor: You also have Alzheimer's disease. In about one year you will forget everything I told you anyway...

(elderly = ältere/r; thorough = gründlich; examination = Untersuchung; news = Neuigkeiten; to estimate = schätzen; awful = furchtbar; be over = hier: vorbei sein; anyway = ohnehin, sowieso)

12 MEDICAL HISTORY

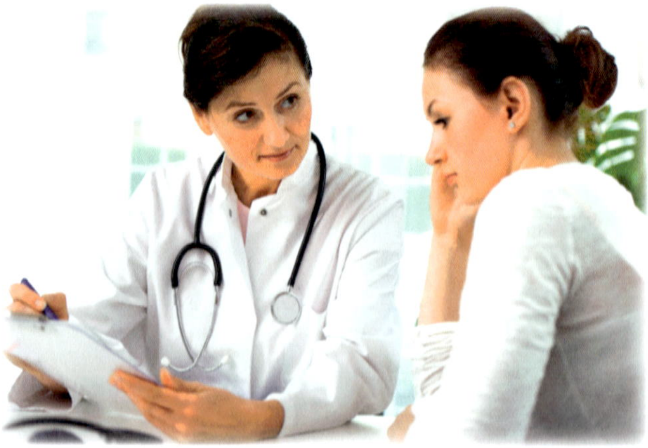

Before a doctor starts treating a patient who he or she does not know very well, it is advisable to ask the patient questions about previous or still persisting diseases, allergies or other medical conditions. These may have an effect on a patient's medical treatment or the medication that the doctor prescribes. The questionnaire below serves as a source of information on the medical history of a patient. A qualified medical employee should understand all the words in this questionnaire.

Dear patient

Diseases of any kind may have an effect on medical treatment. For this reason you are kindly requested to complete this questionnaire. It will be attached to your patient's file and mainly serves to adjust our medical treatment to your state of health.

Patient's name:	Family doctor's name:
Date of birth:	Family doctor's address:
Telephone/home:	Name of patient's health insurance company:
Employer:	Insured person's name: (if different from patient's name)
Occupation:	Insured person's address (zip code, town/place, and street):
Employer's address:	Telephone/work:

Medical history

1. Do you suffer from high blood pressure? Yes/No
2. Do you suffer from low blood pressure? Yes/No
3. Do you suffer from hyperthyroidism? Yes/No
4. Do you suffer from hypothyroidism? Yes/No
5. Do/Did you have a heart disease? Yes/No
   - Heart insuffiency Yes/No
   - Valvular defect Yes/No
   - Endocarditis Yes/No
   - Heart surgery Yes/No
   - Cardiac pacemaker Yes/No
   - Heart pass Yes/No
     issued by: ....
6. Do/Did you suffer from any of the following diseases?
   - Diabetes Yes/No
   - Blood diseases (e.g. clotting disorder) Yes/No
   - Allergies (e.g. hay fever) Yes/No
   - Asthma/lung diseases Yes/No
   - Diseases of the nervous system Yes/No
   - Liver disease/Icterus(Jaundice) Yes/No
   - Rheumatism/Rheumatic fever Yes/No
   - Kidney disease Yes/No
   - Epilepsy Yes/No
   - Stomach/Intestinal disease Yes/No
   - Immune deficiency (HIV) Yes/No
7. Do you take anticoagulants (blood thinners)? Yes/No
8. Are you allergic to certain medication? Yes/No
   If yes, which? ....
9. Are you suffering from any other diseases? Yes/No
   If yes, which? ....
10. What medication are you taking at the present time?

11. When were you X-rayed last?
    Approximate date .... Organs ....
12. Are you pregnant? Yes/No
13. Do you wish to get local anaesthesia? Yes/No
14. Have you been at hospital or have you received medical treatment during the past two years? Yes/No

Patient's signature/Date:

Please note:

Even local anaesthesia may affect your ability to drive. Please, drive carefully or even better, have someone else drive you.

Doctor:	Have you ever had trouble with diarrhoea?
Patient:	Yes, but only once.
Doctor:	When was that?
Patient:	When I was at school and the teacher asked me to spell it.

(trouble with = ein Problem mit; diarrhoea = Durchfall; once = ein Mal; ask = hier: bitten; spell = buchstabieren)

ACTIVITY 1

This text contains a lot of new vocabulary. Find the English expressions in the text and add the words to your personal vocabulary list!

Anamnese	es wäre ratsam	vorhergehende/frühere
noch andauernd/bestehend	eine Auswirkung haben auf	Medikation/Arznei
verschreiben	ein Fragebogen	er dient

als Informationsquelle	Information über etwas	Krankheiten jeder Art
medizinische Behandlung	aus diesem Grund	Sie werden höflich gebeten
etwas ausfüllen	er wird beigefügt	die Patientenakte
er dient hauptsächlich dazu	anpassen	Gesundheitszustand
Arbeitgeber	versicherte Person	Postleitzahl
Stadt/Ort	leiden an	Bluthochdruck, Hypertonus
Hypotonus	Schilddrüsenüberfunktion	Schilddrüsenunterfunktion
Herzerkrankung	Herzinsuffizienz	Herzklappenfehler
Endokarditis	Herz-OP	Herzschrittmacher
Schrittmacherpass	ausgestellt durch/von	Blutkrankheit
Gerinnungsstörung	Erkrankung der Lunge	Nervenkrankheit
Lebererkrankung	Ikterus, Gelbsucht	Rheuma
rheumatisches Fieber	Nierenerkrankung	Epilepsie
Magenerkrankung	Darmerkrankung	Immunschwäche
Blutverdünnende Medikamente, Antikoagulanzien	Allergie auf bestimmte Medikamente	zurzeit, momentan
geröntgt	ungefähres Datum	Organe
schwanger sein	örtliche Betäubung, Lokalanästhesie	medizinische Behandlung erhalten
die vergangenen zwei Jahre	Unterschrift	wichtiger Hinweis
beeinträchtigen	die Fahrtüchtigkeit	Fahren Sie vorsichtig!

ACTIVITY 2

Exercise the new words by doing this translation!

1. Ich habe ein paar Fragen über frühere oder noch bestehende Erkrankungen.
2. Noch bestehende Erkrankungen haben eine Auswirkung auf die medizinische Behandlung oder Arzneimittel, die der Arzt verschreibt.
3. Sie werden freundlich gebeten, diesen Fragebogen auszufüllen.
4. Wir legen ihn Ihrer Patientenakte bei.
5. Wir passen unsere Behandlung Ihrem Gesundheitszustand an.
6. Könnten Sie mir den Namen Ihres Arbeitgebers nennen?
7. Welchen Beruf üben Sie aus?
8. Wer ist Ihr Hausarzt?
9. Wie heißt Ihre Krankenversicherung?
10. Leiden Sie an Hypertonus?
11. Leiden Sie an Hypotonie?
12. Haben Sie eine Herzinsuffizienz?
13. Haben Sie einen Herzschrittmacher?

14. Von wem wurde Ihr Schrittmacherpass ausgestellt?
15. Hatten Sie schon einmal eine Endokarditis?
16. Wurde bei Ihnen schon einmal eine Herz-OP durchgeführt?
17. Leiden Sie an einem Herzklappenfehler?
18. Der Patient hat eine Nierenerkrankung.
19. Einige Patienten leiden an einer Gerinnungsstörung.
20. Ich leide an einer Nervenkrankheit.
21. Gelbsucht ist eine Erkrankung der Leber. Ärzte nennen sie auch „Ikterus".
22. Haben Sie eine Magen- oder Darmerkrankung?
23. Nehmen Sie gerinnungshemmende Medikamente?
24. Reagieren Sie allergisch auf bestimmte Medikamente?
25. Sind Sie schwanger?
26. Wünschen Sie eine lokale Betäubung?
27. Wann wurden Sie zuletzt geröntgt?
28. Welche Medikamente nehmen Sie zurzeit?
29. Fahren Sie bitte vorsichtig!

>>> ACTIVITY 3 >>>

A new, only English speaking patient is visiting your surgery. Ask him/her questions about his/her medical history!

1. Klären Sie ihn/sie zunächst darüber auf, warum vor der Behandlung eine Anamnese durch den Arzt wichtig ist.
2. Fragen Sie nach Namen, Geburtsdatum, Telefonnummer und Wohnort (PLZ, Ort, Strasse).
3. Fragen Sie ihn/sie, wo er/sie beschäftigt ist (Name des Arbeitgebers), und welchen Beruf er/sie ausübt.
4. Erkundigen Sie sich nach seinem/ihrem Hausarzt und nach seiner/ihrer KV.
5. Fragen Sie, ob er/sie schon einmal eine Herz-OP hatte.
6. Fragen Sie ob er/sie ...
   - einen Herzschrittmacher hat,
   - einen Schrittmacherpass besitzt,
   - an einer Endokarditis leidet oder an einem Herzklappenfehler.
   - an einer Herzinsuffizienz leidet.
7. Fragen Sie den Patienten/die Patientin, ob er/sie an Diabetes leidet.
8. Fragen Sie, ob er/sie an Bluthochdruck oder niedrigem Blutdruck leidet.
9. Fragen Sie, ob er/sie an irgendwelchen Blutkrankheiten wie z.B. einer Gerinnungsstörung leidet.
10. Fragen Sie, ob er/sie an irgendwelchen Allergien oder Asthma leidet.
11. Fragen Sie, ob er/sie zurzeit blutverdünnende Medikamente oder andere Medikamente nimmt.
12. Fragen Sie, ob er/sie an einer Erkrankung der Nieren oder einer Magen-Darm-Erkankung leidet.
13. Fragen Sie, wann er/sie zuletzt geröntgt wurde.
14. Fragen Sie, ob er/sie örtliche Betäubung wünscht.

EXTENDED VOCABULARY LIST	
ability	Fähigkeit, Begabung
adjust to	anpassen, einstellen auf
affect	beeinträchtigen, beeinflussen
anaesthesia **local anaesthesia** **general anaesthesia**	Narkose, Anästhesie, Betäubung lokale Betäubung, Lokalanästhesie Vollnarkose
anticoagulant	gerinnungshemmendes Mittel
approximate(ly)	ungefähr, annähernd
attach to	beilegen, beifügen, als Anlage beilegen
cardiac	Herz-
clot	Klümpchen, Blutgerinnsel, gerinnen (lassen)
clotting, coagulation	Gerinnung
coagulate, clot	gerinnen
date	Datum, Zeitpunkt, Verabredung
defect	Fehler, Schaden, Defekt
effect on	Auswirkung auf, sich auf etwas auswirken
endocarditis	Endokarditis, Herzinnenhautentzündung
family doctor/physician	Hausarzt
file	Akte, Aktenordner, Feile, ablegen
health/medical insurance	Krankenversicherung
heart insufficiency	ungenügende Herzleistung, Herzleistungsstörung
insufficiency	Mangel, Insuffizienz
insufficient	unzulänglich, ungenügend
insured	versichert
issue	Frage, Problem, Ausgabe, ausgeben, ausstellen, herausgeben
kind	herzlich, freudlich, entgegenkommend, Art, Gattung
kindly	freundlicherweise
local	lokal, örtlich, ortsansässig, hiesig

EXTENDED VOCABULARY LIST	
medical condition	Beschwerden, Krankheiten, Erkrankungen, state of health
note	Notiz
notice	Hinweis, bemerken
other	andere/s
pace	Schritt, Gangart, Tempo
pacemaker	Schrittmacher
past	vergangen, beendet, ehemalig, früher, Vergangenheit
persist (in)	andauern, fortbestehen, bestehen auf, nicht nachgeben
persisting	anhaltend, noch andauernd
place	Ort, Gemeinde, platzieren
pregnant	schwanger, trächtig, bedeutungsvoll
present	momentan, gegenwärtig
previous	früher, vorhergehend
receive	erhalten, empfangen
request	Bitte, bitten
serve as	dienen als
state	Zustand, Staat
surgery	Operation
valve	Ventil, Klappe
valvular defect	(Herz-)Klappenfehler
zip code (US), postal code (Brit.)	Postleitzahl

Never forget:

A joke a day keeps the doctor away!

(joke = Witz; a day = pro Tag; to keep away = fernhalten)

A–Z WORD LIST

English	German
abroad	im Ausland
accident	Unfall, Zufall
accompanied	begleitet von
ache	Schmerz
address	Adresse
adjust	anpassen
administration	Verwaltung
advice	Rat(schlag)
advisable	ratsam
advise	raten
allow	erlauben
anaesthetic	Anästhetikum
analgesic	Analgetikum
animal hair	Tierhaare
antibiotic	Antibiotikum
anticoagulant	Antikoagulanz
anything	irgend etwas
appointment	Termin
approximately	ungefähr
assist	helfen, assistieren
assistant	Helfer/in, Assistent/in
assume	annehmen
at all	überhaupt
at least	mindestens
attach	hinzufügen
aware (of)	bewusst
back	Rücken, Rückseite
back home	zuhause
bacteria	Bakterien
bad	schlimm, schlecht
bad luck	Pech
benign	gutartig
better off	besser dran
bladder	Blase
blocked	verstopft
bone	Knochen

English	German
bowels	Eingeweide, Darm
box	Schachtel
break	Bruch, Pause
breathing	Atmung
bruised	gequetscht
busy	arbeitsreich, beschäftigt
by now	bis jetzt
Bye!	Tschüss
cancer	Krebs
capsule	Kapsel
card reader	Kartenlesegerät
cardiologist	Kardiologe
cash	Bargeld
catch	fangen, verstehen
cause	Ursache, verursachen
centigrade	Celsius-Grad
certain	sicher
certainly	sicherlich
charge	Gebühr, berechnen
chat	Gespräch
check-up	Untersuchung
chemist	Apotheker
chemist's shop	Apotheke (Brit.)
chest-pain	Brustschmerz
Christian name	Vorname, Taufname
circulation	Kreislauf
circulatory trouble	Kreislaufproblem
clinical	klinisch
cold	Erkältung, Kälte, kalt
colleague	Kollege
college	Fachhochschule
complete	vollständig
construction	Bau, Konstruktion
consult	aufsuchen, beraten
consultant	Berater, hier: Facharzt
contact lense	Kontaktlinse

English	German
corridor	Flur
coughing	Husten
couple	paar, Paar
cover	hier: abdecken
crossroads	Kreuzung
current	laufend
cut	Schnitt(wunde)
cyst	Zyste
decide	entscheiden
defect	Schaden, Defekt
degree	Grad
dermatologist	Hautarzt
diarrhoea	Durchfall
disappear	verschwinden
disc	Scheibe
disease	Erkrankung
disorder	Störung
disturb	stören
dosage	Dosierung
draw up	entwerfen
drawer	Schublade
dress	verbinden, anziehen
drops	Tropfen
each	jede/r/s einzelne
effect	Auswirkung
efficient	wirksam
employed by	beschäftigt bei
employee	Arbeitnehmer
employer	Arbeitgeber
empty stomach	nüchtern (leerer Magen)
enter	betreten
entire	gesamt
equipment	Ausstattung
especially	besonders
essential	wesentlich, essentiell
expect	erwarten
experienced	erfahren, versiert
expression	Ausdruck
extended	erweitert

English	German
fact	Tatsache
family doctor	Hausarzt
family name	Familienname
famous	sehr bekannt, berühmt
fee	Gebühr
feverish	fiebrig
few	wenige
fill in	ausfüllen, einfüllen
flu	Influenza, Grippe
flu bug	Grippebazillus
flu-like	grippeähnlich
flyer	Faltblatt, Flugblatt, Flyer
form	Formular, Form
forrest	größerer Wald
frequent/ly	häufig
further	weiter, weitergehend
gall bladder	Gallenblase
general	allgemein
glad	froh
glasses	Brille
ground	Boden
grow worse	schlimmer werden
guess	raten, annehmen
hang on	warten, dran bleiben
harmful	schädlich
harmless	unschädlich
hay fever	Heuschnupfen
health insurance	Krankenkasse
hesitate	zögern
history	Vorgeschichte
hold on	warten
How come?	Wieso? Wodurch?
however	jedoch
hyperthyroidism	Hyperthyreose
hypothyroidism	Hypothyreose
immune deficiency	Immunschwäche
in advance	im Voraus
infected	infiziert
injection	Injektion

English	German
injured	verletzt
injury	Verletzung
instruction	Anleitung
insufficiency	Insuffizienz
insured	versichert
internal	inner/e/s
intestines	Darm, Eingeweide
iron bar	Eisenstange
issue	ausstellen
itchy	juckend
jammed	eingeklemmt
jaundice	Gelbsucht
kidney	Niere
kind	herzlich
knee	Knie
laboratory, lab	Labor
lately	neulich, kürzlich
leave	lassen, hinterlassen
lecture	Vortrag, Vorlesung
lecturer	Dozent
liver	Leber
local	ortsansässig
lose	verlieren
lump	Geschwulst, Knoten
mainly	hauptsächlich
malignant	bösartig, maligne
married	verheiratet
meadow	Wiese
meal	Mahlzeit
mean	bedeuten, meinen
measure	messen, Maß
medical	medizinisch
medical card	KV-karte
medication	Medikation
meniscus	Meniskus
message	Mitteilung, Nachricht
might	könnte vielleicht
mild	mild, gering
mixture	Mixtur

English	German
move	umziehen, bewegen
nasal spray	Nasenspray
nationality	Staatsangehörigkeit
nerve	Nerv
nervous system	Nervensystem
neurologist	Neurologe
next door	gleich nebenan
none	kein/e/er/es
note	Notiz
notice	Anmerkung, Hinweis
now and then	hin und wieder
obligation	Verpflichtung
occupation	Beschäftigung
off-duty	dienstfrei
opportunity	Gelegenheit
oculist	Augenarzt
organ	Organ, Orgel
orthopaedist	Orthopäde
outside	draußen, außerhalb
over there	drüben
pacemaker	Schrittmacher
paediatrician	Kinderarzt/ärztin
pain	Schmerz
pain-killer	Schmerzstiller
painkilling	schmerzstillend
pancreas	Bauchspeicheldrüse
part	Teil, Rolle
patient´s file	Patientenakte
payment	Zahlung
persist	andauern
personal	persönlich, intim
pharmacy	Apotheke (US)
pill	Pille
place	platzieren, abstellen, Ort
pluck	pflücken
pollen	Pollen
poor	schlecht, arm
postal code	Postleitzahl (Brit.)

English	German
pregnant	schwanger
prescription	Rezept, Verschreibung
presently	momentan, zurzeit
previous	vorhergehend
profession	Beruf
professional	beruflich, professionell
provider	Versorger, Anbieter
put down	niederschreiben
put through	verbinden, durchstellen
questionnaire	Fragebogen
radiologist	Radiologe
rare	selten
ray	Strahl
reason	Grund
receive	erhalten
reception	Anmeldung, Empfang
record card	Karteikarte
refer	überweisen
relieve	erleichtern
request	erbitten
rheumatism	Rheuma
ring	anrufen, Ring
sample	Muster, Probe
scan	abtasten (Oberfläche)
seat	Sitzplatz, Sitz
self-medication	Selbstmedikation
sensible	vernünftig
sensitive	empfindlich
serious	ernst
serve	dienen
several	verschiedene
sharp	scharf, stechend
sickness	Übelkeit
side effect	Nebenwirkung
sign	unterschreiben, Zeichen
signature	Unterschrift
sleeve	Ärmel
slip	rutschen
sneezing	Niesen
so far	bisher
soon	bald
sore	entzündet
source	Quelle
specialized	spezialisiert
specimen	Probe, Muster
spread	ausbreiten
spring	Frühling
staff	Personal
stand	hier: aushalten
stand for	stehen für
state of health	Gesundheitszustand
stiff	steif
stitch	nähen
stomach	Magen
suffer from	leiden an
sure	sicher, klar
Sure!	Na klar!
surgeon	Chirurg
surgery	Operation, Praxis
surgical	chirurgisch
surname	Nachname
survey	Umfrage, Übersicht
survive	überleben
swallow	schlucken
tablet	Tablette
take	nehmen, ergreifen
take care (of)	sich kümmern (um)
take off	ablegen (Kleidung)
take out	hier: abschließen
technique	Methode, Verfahren
technology	Technik, Technologie
throat	Hals, Kehle, Rachen
thyroid gland	Schilddrüse
tick	hier: Zecke
topic	Thema
treatment	Behandlung
ultrasound	Ultraschall
ultrasound scan	Ultraschalluntersuchung

English	German
update	erneuern/Erneuerung
urgent	dringend
urine specimen	Urinprobe
urological	urologisch
urologist	Urologe
urology	Urologie
vaccinate	impfen
vaccination	Impfung
vomit	erbrechen
waste	Abfall, Verschwendung
watery	wässrig
well-known	gut bekannt
wheezing	Keuchen
while	während, Weile
wonder	sich fragen
work	wirken, arbeiten
workmate	Arbeitskollege
worse	schlimmer
wound	Wunde
X-ray	Röntgen
zip code (US); postal code (UK)	Postleitzahl

German	English
Abfall, Verschwendung	waste
ablegen (Kleidung)	take off
abdecken	cover
abschließen (Versicherung)	take out
abtasten (Oberfläche)	scan
Adresse	address
allgemein	general
Analgetikum	analgesic
Anästhetikum	anaesthetic
andauern	persist
Anleitung	instruction
Anmeldung, Empfang	reception
Anmerkung, Hinweis	notice
annehmen	assume
anpassen	adjust
anrufen, Ring	ring
Antibiotikum	antibiotic
Antikoagulanz	anticoagulant
Apotheke (UK)	chemist´s shop
Apotheke (US)	pharmacy
Apotheker	chemist/pharmacyst
Arbeitgeber	employer
Arbeitnehmer	employee
Arbeitskollege	workmate
arbeitsreich, beschäftigt	busy
Ärmel	sleeve
Atmung	breathing
aushalten	stand
aufsuchen, beraten	consult
Augenarzt	oculist
ausbreiten	spread
Ausdruck	expression
ausfüllen, einfüllen	fill in

German	English
Ausstattung	equipment
ausstellen	issue
Auswirkung	effect
Bakterien	bacteria
bald	soon
Bargeld	cash
Bau, Konstruktion	construction
Bauchspreicheldrüse, Pankreas	pancreas
bedeuten, meinen	mean
begleitet von	accompanied
Behandlung	treatment
Berater, hier: Facharzt	consultant
Beruf	profession
beruflich, professionell	professional
beschäftigt bei	employed by
Beschäftigung	occupation
besonders	especially
besser dran	better off
betreten	enter
bewusst	aware (of)
bis jetzt	by now
bisher	so far
Blase	bladder
Blutprobe	blood specimen
Boden	ground
bösartig, maligne	malignant
Brille	glasses
Bruch, Pause	break
Brustschmerz	chest-pain
Celsius-Grad	centigrade
Chirurg	surgeon
chirurgisch	surgical
Darm, Eingeweide	intestines
dienen	serve
dienstfrei	off-duty
Dosierung	dosage

German	English
Dozent	lecturer
draußen, außerhalb	outside
dringend	urgent
drüben	over there
Durchfall	diarrhoea
eingeklemmt	jammed
Eingeweide, Darm	bowels
Eisenstange	iron bar
empfindlich	sensitive
entscheiden	decide
entwerfen	draw up
entzündet	sore
erbitten	request
erbrechen	vomit
erfahren, versiert	experienced
erhalten	receive
Erkältung, Kälte, kalt	cold
Erkrankung	disease
erlauben	allow
erleichtern	relieve
erneuern/Erneuerung	update
ernst	serious
erwarten	expect
erweitert	extended
Fachhochschule	college
Faltblatt, Flugblatt	flyer
Familienname	family name
fangen, verstehen	catch
fiebrig	feverish
Flur	corridor
Formular, Form	form
Fragebogen	questionnaire
froh	glad
Frühling	spring
Gallenblase	gall bladder
Gebühr	fee, charge
Gelbsucht	jaundice

German	English
Gelegenheit	opportunity
gequetscht, gestaucht	bruised
gesamt	entire
Geschwulst, Knoten	lump
Gespräch	chat
Gesundheitszustand	state of health
gleich nebenan	next door
Grad	degree
grippeähnlich	flu-like
Grippebazillus	flu bug
größerer Wald	forrest
Grund	reason
gut bekannt	well-known
gutartig	benign
Hals, Kehle, Rachen	throat
häufig	frequent/ly
hauptsächlich	mainly
Hausarzt	family doctor
Hautarzt	dermatologist
helfen, assistieren	assist
Helfer/in, Assistent/in	assistant
herzlich	kind
Heuschnupfen	hay fever
hin und wieder	now and then
hinzufügen	attach
Husten	coughing
Hyperthyreose	hyperthyroidism
Hypothyreose	hypothyroidism
im Ausland	abroad
im Voraus	in advance
Immunschwäche	immune deficiency
impfen	vaccinate
Impfung	vaccination
infiziert	infected
Influenza, Grippe	flu
Injektion	injection
inner/e/s	internal

German	English
irgend etwas	anything
jede/r/s einzelne	each
jedoch	however
juckend	itchy
Kapsel	capsule
Karteikarte	record card/file card
Kartenlesegerät	card reader
kein/e/er/es	none
Keuchen	wheezing
Kinderarzt/ärztin	paediatrician
klinisch	clinical
Knie	knee
Knochen	bone
Kollege	colleague
könnte vielleicht	might
Kontaktlinse	contact lense
Krankenkasse	health insurance
Krebs	cancer
Kreislauf	circulation
Kreislaufproblem	circulatory trouble
Kreuzung	crossroads
KV-karte	medical card
Labor	laboratory, lab
lassen, hinterlassen	leave
laufend, aktuell	current
Leber	liver
leiden an	suffer from
Magen	stomach
Mahlzeit	meal
Medikation	medication
medizinisch	medical
Meniskus	meniscus
messen, Maß	measure
Methode, Verfahren	technique
mild, gering	mild
mindestens	at least
Mitteilung, Nachricht	message
Mixtur	mixture
momentan, zurzeit	presently
Muster, Probe	specimen, sample
Na klar!	Sure!
Nachname	surname
nähen	stitch
Nasenspray	nasal spray
Nebenwirkung	side effect
nehmen, ergreifen	take
Nerv	nerve
Nervensystem	nervous system
neulich, kürzlich	lately
Neurologe	neurologist
niederschreiben	put down
Niere	kidney
Niesen	sneezing
Notiz	note
nüchtern (leerer Magen)	empty stomach
Operation, Praxis	surgery
Organ, Orgel	organ
Ort	place
Orthopäde	orthopaedist
ortsansässig, lokal	local
paar, Paar	couple
Patientenakte	patient´s file
Pech	bad luck
Personal	staff
persönlich, intim	personal
pflücken	pluck
Pille	pill
platzieren, abstellen	place
Pollen	pollen
Postleitzahl (Brit.)	postal code
Postleitzahl (US)	zip code
Quelle	source
Radiologe	radiologist
Rat(schlag)	advice
raten	advise
raten, annehmen	guess

German	English
ratsam	advisable
Rezept, Verschreibung	prescription
Rheuma	rheumatism
Röntgen	X-ray
Rücken, Rückseite	back
rutschen	slip
Schachtel	box
Schaden, Defekt	defect
schädlich	harmful
scharf, stechend	sharp
Scheibe	disc
Schilddrüse	thyroid gland
schlecht, arm	poor
schlimm, schlecht	bad
schlimmer	worse
schlimmer werden	grow worse
schlucken	swallow
Schmerz	ache, pain
schmerzstillend	painkilling
Schmerzstiller	pain-killer
Schnitt(wunde)	cut
Schrittmacher	pacemaker
Schublade	drawer
schwanger	pregnant
sehr bekannt, berühmt	famous
Selbstmedikation	self-medication
selten	rare
sich fragen	wonder
sich kümmern (um)	take care (of)
sicher	certain
sicher, klar	sure
sicherlich	certainly
Sitzplatz, Sitz	seat
spezialisiert	specialized
Staatsangehörigkeit	nationality
stehen für	stand for
steif	stiff
stören	disturb
Störung	disorder
Strahl	ray
Stuhlprobe	stool specimen
Tablette	tablet
Tatsache	fact
Technik	technology
Teil, Rolle	part
Termin	appointment
Thema	topic
Tierhaare	animal hair
Tropfen	drops
Tschüss	Bye!
Übelkeit	sickness
Umfrage, Übersicht	survey
überhaupt	at all
überleben	survive
überweisen	refer
Ultraschall	ultrasound
Ultraschalluntersuchung	ultrasound scan
umziehen, bewegen	move
Unfall, Zufall	accident
ungefähr	approximately
unschädlich	harmless
unterschreiben, Zeichen	sign
Unterschrift	signature
Untersuchung	check-up
Urinprobe	urine specimen
Urologe	urologist
Urologie	urology
urologisch	urological
Ursache, verursachen	cause
verbinden, anziehen	dress
verbinden, durchstellen	put through
verheiratet	married

German	English
verletzt	injured
Verletzung	injury
verlieren	lose
vernünftig	sensible
Verpflichtung	obligation
verschiedene	several
verschwinden	disappear
versichert	insured
Versorger, Anbieterr	provide
verstopft	blocked
Verwaltung	administration
vollständig	complete
Vorgeschichte	history
vorhergehend	previous
Vorname, Taufname	Christian name
Vortrag, Vorlesung	lecture
während, Weile	while
warten	hold on

German	English
warten, dran bleiben	hang on
wässrig	watery
weiter, weitergehend	further
wenige	few
wesentlich, essentiell	essential
Wiese	meadow
Wieso? Wodurch?	How come?
wirken, arbeiten	work
wirksam	efficient
Wunde	wound
Zahlung	payment
Zecke	tick
zögern	hesitate
zuhause	back home
Zyste	cyst